Guiding Neurosurgery by Evidence

Progress in Neurological Surgery

Vol. 19

Series Editor

L. Dade Lunsford *Pittsburgh, Pa.*

KARGER

Guiding Neurosurgery by Evidence

Volume Editor

Bruce E. Pollock *Rochester, Minn.*

6 figures and 23 tables, 2006

KARGER

Basel · Freiburg · Paris · London · New York ·
Bangalore · Bangkok · Singapore · Tokyo · Sydney

Bruce E. Pollock, MD
Department of Neurological Surgery, Mayo Clinic
200 First Street SW
Rochester, Minn., USA

Library of Congress Cataloging-in-Publication Data
Guiding neurosurgery by evidence / volume editor Bruce
E. Pollock.
p. ; cm. – (Progress in neurological surgery,
ISSN 0079-6492 ; v.
19)
Includes bibliographical references and index.
ISBN 3-8055-8130-0 (hard cover : alk. paper)
1. Nervous system–Surgery. 2. Evidence-based
medicine. I. Pollock,
Bruce E. II. Series.
[DNLM: 1. Neurosurgical Procedures. 2. Evidence-
Based Medicine. W1
PR673 v.19 2006 / WL 368 G947 2006]
RD593.G85 2006
617.4′8–dc22
2006013728

Bibliographic Indices. This publication is listed in bibliographic services, including Current Contents® and Index Medicus.

Disclaimer. The statements, options and data contained in this publication are solely those of the individual authors and contributors and not of the publisher and the editor(s). The appearance of advertisements in the book is not a warranty, endorsement, or approval of the products or services advertised or of their effectiveness, quality or safety. The publisher and the editor(s) disclaim responsibility for any injury to persons or property resulting from any ideas, methods, instructions or products referred to in the content or advertisements.

Drug Dosage. The authors and the publisher have exerted every effort to ensure that drug selection and dosage set forth in this text are in accord with current recommendations and practice at the time of publication. However, in view of ongoing research, changes in government regulations, and the constant flow of information relating to drug therapy and drug reactions, the reader is urged to check the package insert for each drug for any change in indications and dosage and for added warnings and precautions. This is particularly important when the recommended agent is a new and/or infrequently employed drug.

www.karger.com
Printed in Switzerland on acid-free paper by Reinhardt Druck, Basel
ISSN 0079–6492
ISBN-10: 3–8055–8130–0
ISBN-13: 978–3–8055–8130–1

To Kristen, for whom all the evidence shows
how lucky I am to share my life with her.

Contents

Series Editor's Note

I am indebted to Bruce Pollock for agreeing to sponsor this superb text on evidence-based medicine as it applies to the field of neurological surgery. Dr. Pollock has put together a tremendous team of experts, and the enclosed volume should be must reading for all neurosurgeons as well as trainees. We all try to practice some form of evidence-based medicine. We all try to resist at the same time the concept of cookbook medicine. In a series of well-documented and erudite chapters beginning with Dr. Mark Linskey, the authors outline the pros and cons of an evidence-based medicine approach. Primary foci include brain tumors, pediatric neurosurgery, cerebrovascular and endovascular surgery, spine disease, radiosurgery, traumatic brain injury, and chronic pain management. These chapters cover a large component of modern-day neurosurgery. The authors rightfully show the potential value of evidence-based medicine while emphasizing the absence of a clear-cut prospective documentation that the application of its principles has a measurable impact on the delivery of medical care for individual patients or populations at large. Neurosurgeons, however, must take note of the many recent advances in health care delivery and technology, and strive to understand the rationale of current procedures and approaches. A commitment to understanding evidence-based medicine helps.

L. Dade Lunsford, MD

Preface

The history of medicine is marked by a series of important changes that have advanced its science and benefited patients worldwide. Progress is notable in our understanding of a vast array of pathologic states, the medical and surgical treatment of these diseases, and innovative technologies that constantly permit patients to be managed more effectively. Despite the significant changes that have occurred in our delivery of medical care, for the most part, medical decision making has been rooted in the subjective opinions of individual or groups of physicians based largely on local traditions and anecdotal experience. Evidence-based medicine (EBM) arose as a philosophical alternative to this dogmatic approach to medical care, and has attempted to reduce the importance of intuition and unsystematic clinical experience to permit a more detached, objective basis for clinical decision making. The field of EBM has developed from the 1970s until the present due to advancements in epidemiology, biostatistics, and information technology. The science of EBM recognizes that the quality of data in the medical literature can be ranked with information derived from randomized clinical trials (RCT) having the greatest validity, and that lower sources of information need to be assessed based on the rules of evidence. When multiple RCTs are available and all provide the same conclusion, then guidelines can be developed to assist physicians about appropriate health care for individual patients. In practice, EBM defines the question of interest, guides a search of the appropriate medical literature, aids in a critical methodological assessment of the data available, and then applies these findings to aid in diagnosis and treatment of patients.

The field of neurological surgery takes great pride in the development and incorporation of novel technologies allowing the treatment of a wide variety of conditions including cerebrovascular disease, neuro-oncology, spinal pathologies, and functional disorders. However, the exponential growth of information that must be deciphered by each practicing neurosurgeon makes it incumbent that they learn the basic methods of EBM so that they can effectively prioritize the published literature and condense its contents into a more understandable and useful form. Yet, despite an appreciation that RCT represent the 'gold standard' of medical evidence, a variety of reasons exist that limit the practical ability of neurosurgeons to perform RCTs for each situation. First, and particularly relevant to neurosurgery, is that the condition of interest may be rare. Second, for benign tumors such as meningiomas or vestibular schwannomas, the success of an operation in preventing tumor recurrence or progression may not be evident for 10 or more years after surgery. Thus, the information derived from case series (level 4 evidence) may be the best available data to base clinical decision making for patients with benign tumors and extended life expectancies. Third, few patients are willing to participate in randomized trials in which one group has open surgery whereas the other group is managed by a less invasive method such as endovascular therapy or stereotactic radiosurgery. For these and many other reasons, neurosurgeons most often have to base their daily decision making on rather poor quality evidence.

The goal of this book is to provide a succinct review of contemporary neurosurgical practice when evaluated by EBM standards. The first chapter introduces the reader to the concept and principles of EBM. The subsequent chapters address the topics of brain tumor epidemiology, benign adult brain tumors, pediatric neurosurgery, endovascular treatment of cerebrovascular disorders, lumbar spine surgery, minimally invasive spine surgery, stereotactic radiosurgery, trauma, and the treatment of chronic pain disorders by neurostimulation. Each chapter summarizes the available literature and grades it according to the quality of the evidence. In addition, the book highlights not only the usefulness of EBM in neurosurgical practice, but also its limitations with regard to neurosurgical disorders that are frequently rare and therefore impossible to evaluate in RCTs. It is hoped that this book will be worthwhile for neurological surgeons and neurologists, both practicing physicians and residents in training.

Bruce E. Pollock, MD
Editor

Pollock BE (ed): Guiding Neurosurgery by Evidence.
Prog Neurol Surg. Basel, Karger, 2006, vol 19, pp 1–53

Evidence-Based Medicine for Neurosurgeons: Introduction and Methodology

Mark E. Linskey

Department of Neurological Surgery, University of California, Irvine and UCI Medical Center, Orange, Calif., USA

Abstract

Evidence-based medicine is a tool of considerable value for medicine and neurosurgery that provides a secure base for clinical practice and practice improvement, but is not without inherent drawbacks, weaknesses and limitations. EBM finds answers to only those questions open to its techniques, and the best available evidence can be a far cry from scientific truth. With the support and backing of governmental agencies, professional medical societies, the AAMC, the ACGME, and the ABMS, EBM is likely here to stay. The fact that: (1) EBM philosophy and critical appraisal techniques have become fully integrated into the training and culture of our younger colleagues, (2) that maintenance of certification will require individuals to demonstrate personal evidence based practice based on tracking and critical analysis of personal practice outcomes as part of the performance-based learning and improvement competency, and (3) that the progressively growing national healthcare expenditures will necessitate increasing basis of reimbursement and funding based on evidence-based effectiveness and guidelines, all point to the likelihood that complete immersion of neurosurgical practice in EBM is inevitable. This article thoroughly explores the history of EBM in medicine in general and in neurosurgery in particular. Emphasis is placed on identifying the legislative and regulatory motive forces at work behind its promulgation and the role that organized medicine has taken to facilitate and foster its acceptance and implementation. An accounting of resources open to neurosurgeons, and a detailed description EBM clinical decision-making methodology is presented. Special emphasis is placed on outlining the methodology as well as the limitations of meta-analyses, randomized clinic trials, and clinical practice parameter guidelines. Commonly perceived objections, as well as substantive problems and limitations of EBM assumptions, tools, and approaches both for individual clinical practice and health policy design and implementation are explored in detail.

Background

Four important movements in modern medicine began to converge in the 1970s and gradually came to be called 'evidence-based medicine' (EBM). The first, begun in the 1950s and 1960s and led by a British epidemiologist named Archie Cochrane, was a call to collect, collate, and summarize all data from randomized clinical trials (RCTs) in obstetrics and gynecology in one location for use in clinical decision making. Dr. Cochrane noted that most obstetrics and gynecology physicians were unaware of RCT clinical research results and had not implemented findings into practice, as well as the fact that physicians in the field were continuing to perform RCTs on questions that had already been answered years ago (a data implementation gap) [1]. Dr. Cochrane's efforts led to the first comprehensive database of RCT results in medicine, covering obstetrics. This was expanded in 1992 to include most of medicine and came to be known as the Cochrane Collaboration [2], which published its first CD-ROM of systematic reviews of clinical trials in 1995.

The second movement centered upon advancements in the science of clinical epidemiology, particularly in biostatistics with an emphasis on RCTs. This led to the development of a peer-review literature, evidence-based approach to medical education and learning in the 1970s and 1980s at McMasters University in Canada [3–6]. This effort overlapped with the clinical guidelines development movement in Canada and the US and the clinical outcomes movement in the US in the 1980s [7–13].

The actual term 'evidence-based medicine' was coined at McMasters University in Canada in 1991 [14] and appeared in print for the first time in 1992 [15]. It refers to a philosophical approach towards clinical decision making (EBM) and establishment of healthcare policy (evidence-based healthcare, EBC) that emphasizes original clinical research in the peer-review literature as the source of 'evidence'. It establishes 'rules of evidence' or a hierarchy of strength of evidence based upon analysis of methodological rigor of the published studies, and emphasizes the priority and primacy of data from RCTs and meta-analysis of RCTs in making clinical, guidelines, and healthcare policy decisions regarding therapy.

The development of EBM and its rapid popularization and proliferation from the 1990s through today would not have been possible without significant progress in information technology, electronic literature archiving and indexing, the development of the Internet, as well as embracement of, and investment in, the approach and philosophy by governmental agencies and organized medicine. The National Library of Medicine (NLM) at the National Institute of Health (NIH) in the US began to collect and collate medical literature into a single database in the 1960s. By 1964, the Medical Literature Analysis and Retrieval System

(MEDLARS) became operational. By 1971 online access to a subset of information in MEDLARS became available through MEDLINE. By 1986, the first PC-based user-friendly software for accessing MEDLARS (Grateful Med) was introduced by the NLM. In 1997 free web-based access to MEDLINE via PubMed became available. PubMed is the search software developed by the NLM's National Center for Biotechnology Information. MEDLINE is currently available and searchable at the NLM via free PubMed access or using proprietary subscription MEDLINE software interfaces such as Ovid (Ovid Technologies, New York, N.Y., USA). MEDLINE currently includes citations from as early as 1966, although the early citations often do not have abstracts and are not as well indexed for search purposes. It currently contains citations from more than 4,300 biomedical journals published in the US and in 70 foreign countries.

Description

EBM de-emphasizes intuition, unsystematic clinical experience, and pathophysiologic rationale as sufficient grounds for clinical decision making [15–18]. It emphasizes the skills of problem defining, literature searching, critical methodological assessment and prioritization, and the application of original clinical research findings published in the medical literature to individual clinical and general healthcare decisions [15, 19–22]. Heavily based in clinical epidemiology, EBM divides clinical questions and primary clinical studies into those that address therapy, harm, diagnosis, and prognosis [3, 4]. While editorials, personal commentary, and general review articles are not considered 'studies', and carry no more weight than expert opinion, certain secondary publications are recognized as having impact. Secondary integrative overview publications of evidentiary value include systematic reviews, practice guidelines, decision analysis summaries, and economic analyses (e.g. cost-effective analysis).

For therapeutic questions, EBM insists upon the priority and primacy of data derived from RCTs, particularly when the statistical power of the study is large as a result of being a 'mega-RCT' (>1,000 patients), or a meta-analysis of multiple RCTs. That is not to say that EBM does not recognize non-RCT data, or that RCT data is available for all relevant questions. According to Sackett, EBM is

> 'the conscientious, explicit and judicious use of current best evidence in making decisions about the care of individual patients'. [This involves] 'integrating individual clinical expertise with the best available external clinical evidence from systematic research' [23].

Data from systematic observational non-RCT studies is still evidence; it is just of a lower quality. With EBM, evidence from clinical studies needs to be assessed according to 'rules of evidence' where studies are ranked according to a hierarchy based on the degree of bias inherent in the study design and the degree of methodological rigor of the individual study [21]. EBM requires careful examination of the evidence using a set of formal rules applied in an explicit manner, and then applying the evidence to decision making along with an understanding of the decision-making context and the patient's personal values [24]. There is always evidence, it just may come from the bottom of the hierarchy.

Nonetheless, it is clear that EBM in its purist sense does exclude certain traditional influences on medical decision making and policy making. Common sense inferences, reasoning from basic science pathophysiologic principles in the absence of confirmatory clinical empirical evidence, nonsystematic and nonquantitative summaries of personal experience, and the opinion of 'experts' are all considered suspect and fail to qualify as 'evidence' within the EBM model. Personal and expert opinions are only considered to reach the lowest rung of the EBM evidence rank hierarchy if they are based on an experience that has been systematically tabulated and objectively quantified in such a way that the opinion rendered can be directly supported independently by referral to objectively verifiable data.

Legislative-Regulatory Motive Forces

In the US, government EBM efforts have largely centered around the NIH (through the NLM), the Food and Drug Administration (FDA), and the Department of Health and Human Services (HHS), through the Agency for Healthcare Research and Quality (AHRQ). It is likely only a matter of time before these initiatives are linked to reimbursement priorities through the Center for Medicare and Medicaid Services (CMS – formerly HCFA, also within HHS).

In addition to MEDLINE, the NLM maintains a government-run database and website of clinical trials (ClinicalTrials.gov) primarily as an information resource for patients. Stimulated by a resolution in June 2004 from the American Medical Association (AMA), a move is now underway to introduce legislation that will expand this database and integrate it with the FDA by requiring all drug companies to list the existence of clinical drug trials and their subsequent results in the database [25].

The Agency for Health Care Policy and Research (AHCPR) was established as a Public Health Service agency within the Department of HHS in December 1989 under Public Law 101-239 [26]. It was tasked with promoting quality of healthcare, reducing its cost, improving patient safety, decreasing medical errors, and broadening access to essential services by supporting outcomes studies, and implementing their findings through the dissemination of clinical guidelines [27]. During healthcare reform debate 1993–1994, President Clinton's proposal would have expanded the government's role to include analysis of national outcomes data and the promulgation of resultant guidelines [27, 28]. The Clinton proposal would have established a National Quality Management Program as a public authority for this large scale outcomes analysis repository and oversight effort. Since 1996, with the collapse of the Clinton national healthcare initiative, the AHCPR has largely restricted its activities to funding EBM research and disseminating the reports of the research findings. In 1999 the name of the agency was changed to the AHRQ [29], eliminating the perception of a direct influence on federal healthcare policies.

As of 2004, the agency has a budget of USD 269.9 million, ~80% of which is currently awarded as research grants to the 13 extramural Evidence-Based Practice Centers (EPCs) listed in table 1. The AHRQ maintains the National Guideline Clearinghouse (NGC) for evidence-based clinical practice guidelines in a joint initiative with the AMA and America's Health Insurance Plans (AHIP – formerly the American Association of Health Plans).

In countries which have nationalized health services and centrally managed and rationed healthcare, such as the United Kingdom, the degree of support, investment, and integration of EBM into EBC has been more direct, intrusive, and far-reaching. The National Health Service (NHS) Research and Development initiative under Sir Michael Peckham was launched in 1991 [30]. Under pressure to invest in effective procedures and disinvest in ineffective ones [31, 32], the initiative was designed 'to secure a knowledge-based health service in which clinical, managerial, and policy decisions are based on sound and pertinent information about research findings and scientific developments' [33]. This has led to a new system of management intended to provide quality in healthcare (clinical governance) that explicitly requires that funded medical treatments be evidence-based [34].

In 1999, the NHS launched the National Institute for Clinical Excellence (NICE) which is responsible for providing patients, health professionals and the public with authoritative, robust and reliable evidence-based guidance on current 'best practices' in relation to new and existing health technologies [35]. Since January 2002, the NHS has been obliged to provide funding and resources for health professional-prescribed medicines and treatments recommended by NICE through its technology appraisal work program [36]. The implication is that medicines and treatments not specifically recommended by NICE will only be funded as resources permit at the discretion of each local NHS authority.

NICE is also charged with establishing and maintaining clinical guidelines for the NHS [37]. This effort began in 1999 [38]. The first NICE clinical guideline was published in April 2001. Unlike guidelines published by the US NGC, NICE guidelines are required to resolve the conflict between pre-existing association and stakeholder guidelines and take into consideration cost-effectiveness

Table 1. Evidence-based practice centers (EPCs) receiving federal grants from the agency for healthcare research and quality in order to produce evidence-based clinical guidelines (as of June 2002)

Blue Cross and Blue Shield Association, Technology Evaluation Center (TEC) (in collaboration with Kaiser Permanente) Naomi Aronson, PhD, Executive Director David M. Eddy, MD, PhD, Scientific Advisor	Chicago, Ill. http://www.bcbs.com/tec/index.html
Duke University, Center for Clinical Health Policy Research (CCHPR) David B. Matchar, MD, Co-Director Douglas McCrory, MD, Co-Director	Durham, NC http://www.clinpol.mc.duke.edu/
ECRI – Emergency Care Research Institute Charles Turkelson, PhD, Proj. Manager	Plymouth Meeting, PA http://www.ecri.org/
Johns Hopkins EPC Eric B. Bass, MD, MPH, Director	Baltimore, MD http://www.jhsph.edu/epc
McMasters University EPC Parminder Raina, PhD, Director, EPC	Hamilton, Ontario, Canada http://hiru.mcmaster.ca/epc/
Metaworks, Inc. (1997–2001), now defunct	Boston, Mass.
Oregon, EPC (OHSU, Portland VAMC, and Kaiser Permente collaboration) Mark Helfand, MD, MS, MPH, Director, EPC	Portland, Oreg. http://www.ohsu.edu/epc/
RTI-UNC EPC (Research Triangle Institute and UNC, Chapel Hill collaboration) Kathleen Lohr, PhD, Co-Director, RTI Timothy Carey, MD, MPH, Co-Director, UNC	Chapel Hill, N.C. http://www.rti.org/epc/home.html
Southern California – RAND, EPC (RAND, UCLA, UCSD, USC, Cedars-Sinai Medical Center/ZYNX Health, Children's Hospital Los Angeles collaboration) Paul G. Shekelle, MD, PhD, Director Sally C. Morton, PhD, Co-Director	Santa Monica, Calif. http://www.rand.org/health/epc/
Stanford – UCSF, EPC (Stanford – UCSF collaboration) Douglas K. Owens, MD, MS, Director A. Eugene Washington, MD, MSc, Co-Director	Stanford, Calif. http://healthpolicy.stanford.edu/stanford-ucsf-epc/
Tufts – New England MC, EPC Joseph Lau, MD, Director	Boston, Mass. http://www.nemc.org/dccr/ Evidence-based%20Practice.htm

Table 1. (continued)

University of Alberta, EPC (University of Alberta and Capital Health Authority in Edmonton collaboration) Terry Klassen, MD, MSc, Director	Edmonton, Alberta, Canada http://www.epc.ualberta.ca/index.htm
University of Minnesota, EPC Robert Klane, MD, Director	Minneapolis, Minn. http://evidence.ahc.umn.edu
University of Ottawa, EPC Howard Schachter, PhD, Co-Director David Moher, MSc, Co-Director	Ottawa, Canada http://www.uo-epc.org/index.html
University of Texas HSC, San Antonio, EPC (1997–2001), now defunct	San Antonio, Tex.

[39, 40] and practicality along with clinical effectiveness, prior to acceptance as NICE-sanctioned guidelines. Like the AHRQ in the US, NICE 'subcontracts' the actual guideline generation task to approved collaborating centers. As of 2004, the six collaborating centers are listed in table 2.

In addition, the NHS maintains the Centre for Reviews and Dissemination (CRD) in York, UK. This center is tasked with maintaining and controlling dissemination of information from three databases. The Database of Reviews of Clinical Effectiveness (DARE) is a database of systematic reviews of topics from the literature produced by the CRD in affiliation with the Cochrane Collaboration. The NHS Economic Evaluation Database (EED) is a database of collated economic analyses from the peer-reviewed literature individually quality-assessed by the CRD. The Office of Health Technology Assessment (HTA) Database contains information on healthcare technology assessments and is produced in collaboration with the International Network of Agencies for Health Technology Assessment (INAHTA) Secretariat, based in Sweden. It contains records of ongoing projects being conducted by members of INAHTA as well as publications reporting completed technology assessments carried out by INAHTA members and other health technology assessment organizations. The abstracts in the database are descriptive rather than analytical and do not form critical appraisals of the reports.

From 1994 to July 2002 the Research and Development Initiative of the NHS funded a web-based secondary EBM journal called *Bandolier* focused on EBC. The journal selectively republishes systematic reviews and meta-analyses gleaned from searching MEDLINE and the Cochrane database in edited 'bullet' form (thus the name – 'bandolier' – a string of bullets). Published out of Oxford, this evidence-based secondary journal has continued as a subscription and privately sponsored service since 2002. From May 1999 to March 2001, the NHS sponsored the EBM journal, *Bandolier*, to establish the electronic publication

Table 2. National Institute of Clinical Excellence (NICE) of the National Health Service (NHS) of England and Wales National Collaboration Centres for Researching and Establishing Clinical Guidelines (as of June 2004)

National Collaborating Centre for Acute Care
http://www.nice.org.uk/page.aspx?o=202090
Based: Royal College of Surgeons, London, UK
Jacqueline Dutchak, Director
National Collaborating Centre for Chronic Conditions
http://www.nice.org.uk/page.aspx?o=202075
Based: Royal College of Physicians, London, UK
Jane Ingham, Manager
National Collaborating Centre for Nursing and Supportive Care
http://www.nice.org.uk/page.aspx?o=202059
Based: Royal College of Nursing, Oxford, UK
Liz McInnes, Senior Research and Development Fellow
National Collaborating Centre for Mental Health
http://www.nice.org.uk/page.aspx?o=202067
Based: British Psychological Society and the Royal College of Psychiatrists (Joint)
Catherine Pettinari, Senior Project Manager
National Collaborating Centre for Primary Care
http://www.nice.org.uk/page.aspx?o=202051
Based: Royal College of General Practitioners
Nancy Turbull, Chief Executive
National Collaborating Centre for Woman and Children's Health
http://www.nice.org.uk/page.aspx?o=202042
Based: Royal College of Obstetricians and Gynaecologists
Jane Thomas, Director
National Collaborating Centre for Cancer
http://www.nice.org.uk/page.aspx?o=202083
Based: Velindre NHS Trust, Cardiff, Wales
Dr. Andrew Champion, Centre Manager

'ImpAct' as part of an NHS Learning Network for managers, which was the first journal designed to showcase EBC management and service. As part of the NHS Learning Network, ImpAct catalogued and disseminated stories of individual NHS change projects; however, it never evolved to actually provide its own evidence-based management 'evidence' [41], and was apparently discontinued.

The Role of Organized Medicine

Many national medical professional organizations have participated in the advancement and popularization of EBM and EBC through: (1) their own guidelines' production and approval mechanisms, (2) establishing EBM review processes for national presentations and journal article submissions, (3) publication of EBM manuals and/or resources, and (4) sponsorship of continuing medical education in EBM techniques. Three of them (the American College of Physicians – ACP, the British Medical Association – BMA, and the AMA) have gone even further through sponsorship of secondary EBM journals and/or databases of systematic reviews of clinical trials, and advocacy efforts to influence governmental EBC policies and programs.

The ACP, through its journal, the *Annals of Internal Medicine*, established the first secondary EBM journal in 1991 (called the *ACP Journal Club*) that summarized new publications of high relevance and methodological rigor [42]. This journal reviewed >40 journals in English on topics central to general internal medicine. The *ACP Journal Club*, initially published as a bimonthly supplement to the *Annals of Internal Medicine*, has been an independent publication since November 1994. From 1996 though 2001 [43], the ACP also produced an annual CD-ROM entitled 'Best Evidence', a compendium of reviews from the *ACP Journal Club*, the journal, *Evidence-Based Medicine* (jointly sponsored with the BMA), and *Diagnostic Strategies for Common Medical Problems*. Best Evidence was replaced by ACP Journal Club online service in 2001 [43].

The AMA, through its journal, *Journal of the American Medical Association* (JAMA), over the period of 10 years, sponsored the publication of a series of 25 'user's guides to the medical literature' produced by the Evidence-Based Medicine Working Group [20, 44–75]. Along with the ACP, they also compiled these articles for publication into two manuals [76, 77]. The AMA currently sponsors and maintains the NGC for evidence-based clinical practice guidelines in a joint initiative with the AHRQ and AHIP. They are also actively involved in promoting expansion of the existing government clinical trials database to include all previous and ongoing drug trials [25].

The British Medical Association has been extremely active in developing and promoting EBM and EBC through their publishing arm, the British Medical Journal (BMJ) Publishing Group. The BMJ Publishing Group publishes the EBM secondary journal, *Evidence-Based Medicine*. Originally started in 1996 as a joint initiative with the ACP and jointly edited at McMasters University and at the Centre for Evidence-Based Medicine at Oxford in the UK, the journal 'EBM' took a similar secondary review approach as the *ACP Journal Club* but broadened coverage to include surgery, obstetrics, pediatrics, family medicine and psychiatry, in addition to general internal medicine [16, 78]. Similar to the AMA, the BMJ Publishing Group has also published a compendium of EBM journal articles from the BMJ into a more easily accessible manual [79]. The BMJ Publishing Group also manages their own online EBM secondary source for primary care called 'Clinical Evidence'.

Organized neurosurgery has made efforts in the EBM arena with mixed results. In the mid-1990s, the American Association of Neurological Surgeons (AANS) and the Congress of Neurological Surgeons (CNS) established a Joint Committee on the Assessment of Quality (formerly known as the Quality Assessment Committee) under Robert Florin. This joint committee oversaw four subcommittees, two of which were the Outcomes Committee and the Guidelines Committee.

Attempts at establishing two national neurosurgery outcomes studies (one on intracranial aneurysms and the other on carotid endarterectomy) [80–82] came to naught and were discontinued. Difficulties with inadequate organizational infrastructure and expertise to manage these projects led the AANS to create a joint venture with Outcomes Sciences (Boston, Mass., USA) called Neuro-Knowledge (Boston, Mass., USA), for the purpose of potentially contracting for future neurosurgery outcomes analysis studies [83].

The Joint Committee on Assessment of Quality was dissolved fairly recently. The Outcomes Subcommittee has ceased to exist. The Guidelines Committee has been systematically working with each AANS/CNS joint section to establish guidelines based on diagnosis-specific section priorities. The Guidelines Subcommittee has become two separate committees – the AANS Guidelines Committee within the Science Division of the AANS, and the CNS Guidelines Development Committee. The Department of Education and Practice Management of the AANS maintains a repository of clinical guidelines pertinent to neurosurgical diagnoses at http://www.aans.org/practice/guideliens/aans.asp. The listing includes guidelines from agencies and organizations other than the AANS or CNS, but as of June 2004, this site appeared to be in need of updating.

The Accreditation Council for Graduate Medical Education (ACGME), the Association of American Medical Colleges (AAMC), and the American Board of Medical Specialties (ABMS) have all agreed to establish a core of six competencies for training and assessing physicians. These competencies have profound implications for educational curricula for medical school and residency training, board certification, and maintenance of certification as a life-long educational/recertification process. The ACGME endorsed the six competencies on September 28, 1999, after a review process by an eleven member Outcome Project Advisory Group spanning the period January 1998 through February 1999. The review process was not evidence-based. Implementation for residency training programs was initiated in July 2002. The Group on Educational Affairs (GEA) within the AAMC is currently working on integrating the six competencies into medical school curricula through their Competencies Across the Continuum of Health Education (CACHE) project. The ABMS, including the American Board of Neurological Surgeons (ABNS), have structured their maintenance of certification processes around the same six competencies [84].

One of the six competencies is practice-based learning and improvement. Ideally, this competency is intended as a specific link to EBM through ongoing self-assessment of outcome results for the individual physician linked to empiric analysis of the success or failure of performance improvement efforts. The specifics of realistic and practically achievable requirements and compliance criteria have yet to be completely worked out.

Resources

Many books and manuals have now been published to assist neurosurgeons with establishing an evidence-based practice and instituting an evidence-based approach to teaching and making individual clinical decisions [3, 4, 76, 77, 79, 85–89]. While an introductory chapter to a book cannot hope to serve as a detailed textbook, the reader is invited to explore these referenced works for details and more in-depth descriptions and explanations.

While the books and manuals referenced above are the best place to start, even more detail can be had by exploring original articles published on specific topics within EBM. Examples include:

(1) An introduction to applying the EBM Working Group User's Guides and articles on general EBM theory [16–23, 44, 45]
(2) How to evaluate and use articles about therapy or prevention [45, 46]
(3) How to evaluate and use articles about a diagnostic test [47, 48]
(4) How to evaluate and use articles about harm [49]
(5) How to evaluate and use articles about prognosis [50]
(6) How to evaluate and use an overview article [51]
(7) How to evaluate and use articles about clinical decision analysis and clinical decision rules [52, 53]
(8) How to evaluate and use guidelines or healthcare/treatment recommendations [54–56, 64, 65]
(9) How to evaluate and use articles on health services outcomes or utilization review [57, 58]
(10) How to evaluate and use articles assessing quality of life [59]
(11) How to evaluate and use articles on the economics of practice [40, 60, 61, 90]
(12) How to best apply the EBM Working Group User's Guides and published evidence to the care of a specific patient [62, 69, 73, 75]
(13) How to evaluate and use articles on disease probability for establishing and working through a differential diagnosis [63]
(14) How to evaluate and use articles on the clinical manifestations of a disease to assist with establishing a diagnosis [74]

Table 3. Evidence-based journals (a selected list)

ACP Journal Club (printed and electronic versions)
Bandolier (printed and electronic versions)
Bandolera (authorized Spanish language version of *Bandolier*)
Effective Health Care Bulletins
Effectiveness Matters
Evidence
Evidence Based Health Care
Evidence Based Medicine (printed and electronic versions)
Evidence Based Medicine – Edition Française (auth. French language version of EBM)
Evidence Based Mental Health (printed and electronic versions)
Evidence Based Nursing
Journal of Family Practice POEMs (Patient-Oriented Evidence that Matters)
New Zealand Evidence Based Healthcare Bulletin

(15) How to make maximal effective use of electronic health information resources and computer-based clinical decision support systems [66, 70]

(16) How to assess the applicability applying of drug class effects versus individual drug effect, as well as surrogate endpoints from RCTs [67, 68]

(17) How to evaluate and use qualitative study results [72, 73].

Many additional resources exist. In addition to books, manuals, and individual articles, there are now more than ten peer-reviewed EBM journals in publication (table 3). Websites that serve as a source of EBM information, links to other pertinent and useful websites, sources of EBM tools, repositories of electronic EBM Journals or collections of systematic reviews, and repositories for clinical guidelines abound. A noninclusive and selective listing of pertinent websites with their internet addresses is presented in table 4.

EBM Clinical Decision Methodology

EBM is rooted in five linked ideas: (1) that clinical decisions should be based on best available clinical evidence, (2) that the specific clinical problem of interest should determine the type of evidence sought, (3) that the evidence discovered through searching should be sorted and assessed using epidemiologic and biostatistical criteria in order to identify the best evidence, (4) that the conclusions arrived at should be put into action, and (5) that the result of the decision should be objectively evaluated [21]. There are four basic steps to taking an evidence-based approach: (1) formulizing a clear clinical question from a patient's problem, (2) effectively searching the literature for relevant

Table 4. Internet and World Wide Web EBM resources

Government sites
US Agency for Healthcare Research and Quality (AHRQ)
http://www.ahrq.gov
AHRQ – Evidence-Based Practice Centers for Guidelines Development (n = 13)
(see table 1)
US National Guidelines Clearing House (NGC)
http://www.guideline.gov
US National Library of Medicine (NLM)
http://www.nlm.nih.gov
US NLM – Clinical Trials Registry
http://www.ClinicalTrials.gov
US NLM – PubMed (free MEDLINE search engine)
http://ncbi.nlm.nih.gov/entrez/query.fcgi?tool=cdl&otool=cdlotool
NHS National Institute for Clinical Excellence (NICE)
http://www.nice.org.uk
NICE – National Collaborating Centers for Guidelines Development (n = 6)
(see table 2)
NHS Centre for Reviews and Dissemination [access to 3 databases – Database of Reviews of Clinical Effectiveness (DARE), NHS Economic Evaluation Database (EED), and the Office of Health Technology Assessment (HTA) Database]
http://www.york.ac.uk/inst/crd/aboutcrd.htm

Organized medicine sites (selected)
American College of Physicians (ACP)
(ACP Journal Club Online, ACP Publications)
http://www.acponline.org
American Medical Association (AMA)
(JAMA, AMA Publications)
http://www.ama-assn.org
British Medical Association – British Medical Journal Publishing Group
(EBM, Clinical Evidence, BMJPG Publications)
http://www.bmjpg.com
American Association of Neurological Surgeons (AANS)
http://www.neurosurgerytoday.org
AANS – AANS Repository of Clinical Guidelines
http://www.aans.org/practice/guidelines/aans.asp
Congress of Neurological Surgeons (CNS)
http://www.neurosurgeon.org
AANS/CNS Joint Sections (Individual Links Via)
http://www.neurosurgery.org

Other Internet EBM databases and search resources
ACP Journal Club Online (ACP online EBM Journal)
www.acpjc.org
Bandolier (free electronic journal compilation of EBC summaries, meta-analyses and commentary)
http://www.jr2.ox.ac.uk:80/bandolier

Table 4. (continued)

Clinical Evidence (online BMJ Publishing Group resource updated biannually)
http://www.clinicalevidence.com/ceweb/conditions/index.jsp
Cochrane Collaboration
http://www.cochrane.org/index0.htm
Cochrane Library Subscription [contains 4 searchable databases on CD-ROM updated quarterly – Cochrane Database of Systematic Reviews (CDSR), Database of Reviews of Clinical Effectiveness (DARE), Cochrane Controlled Trials Registry (CCTR), Cochrane Review Methodological Database (CRMD)]
http://www.update-software.com/cochrane/cochrane-frame.html
Evidence-Based Medicine (BMJ Publishing Group EBM Journal available online)
http://ebm.bmjjournals.com/
Evidence-Based Medicine Reviews (EBMR – offered as a subscription though Ovid, combines 4 data bases into one for search purposes – Cochrane Database of Systematic Reviews, Database of Abstracts of Reviews of Effectiveness, ACP Journal Club, and the Cochrane Central Registry of Controlled Trials)
http://www.ovid.com/site/catalog/DataBase/904.jsp?top=2&mid=3&bottom=7&subsection=10
Guidelines International Network (51 member organizations including the WHO from 26 countries, maintains an international guidelines library)
http://www.g-i-n.net
Ovid Technologies (electronic literature search software with access to most systematic review databases normally each requiring a separate subscription)
http://www.ovid.com

Internet EBM web sites with tools and links (see also sites in table 1)
Berkeley Systematic Reviews Group
http://www.medepi.org/meta
Canadian Center for Health Evidence
http://www.cche.net/che/home.asp
Center for Evidence Based Medicine, University of Toronto, Canada
http://www.cebm.utoronto.ca
Center for Evidence Based Medicine, Oxford, UK
http://www.cebm.net
Cochrane Reviewer's Handbook
http://www.update-software.com/ccweb/cochrane/hbook.htm
Evidence-Based Medicine Tool Kit, University of Alberta, Canada
http://www.med.ualberta.ca/ebm/ebm.htm
Health Information Research Unit, McMasters University, Hamilton, Canada
http://hiru.mcmaster.ca
Netting the Evidence, The SCHARR Guide to EBP on the Internet (one of the more comprehensive catalogue of EBC websites and resources)
http://www.shef.ac.uk/scharr/ir/netting
Users' Guide to the Medical Literature (JAMA Series available electronically)
www.cche.net/principles/main.asp

All sites accessed successfully using the web addresses provided July 11, 2004.

clinical articles, (3) evaluating (critically appraising) the evidence for its validity and usefulness, and (4) implementing the findings in clinical practice [22].

In general, Sackett et al. [23] identifies two broad forms of questions: background and foreground. Background questions are general knowledge questions about the patient, the diagnosis or the treatment (i.e. why, what, when, where, who and how?) Foreground questions focus on very specific information needs for decision making. These needs may relate to the patient, the main intervention under consideration, alternative interventions under consideration, or a clinical outcome of interest. It is with the latter type of question that an EBM approach is most likely to have impact. Neurosurgery is an intervention- and action-oriented medical subspecialty. As a result, while decisions regarding prevention and diagnosis (e.g. testing) are important, decisions regarding interventions (that rely on assessments of prognosis and harm) tend to be more interesting and relevant to the majority of our decisions. To benefit both the patient and the clinician, the question must be well built – which means, both relevant to the patient's problem, and phrased in a way that directs the subsequent search to relevant and precise answers [20, 88, 89].

In general, effectively searching the literature for relevant clinical articles has become much faster and more efficient with the use of electronic search engines for the NLM MEDLINE database [66, 70]. On the other hand, searching by hand for clinical studies published in books or book chapters and articles published prior to 1966 has become more difficult and less efficient. Many of us have forgotten where the medical school library is located as we have become more focused and reliant on our desktop computers for search access. Many medical centers have witnessed deterioration in their medical libraries through neglect and funding reductions as the number of library visitors and the need for librarian services diminish. As MEDLINE searches have become common place, many of us have forgotten (or have never been taught!) how to search journal articles using Index Medicus.

Even electronic literature searching is becoming more complicated if comprehensiveness is sought or desired. Many clinical trials, systematic reviews, and other secondary overviews not published in journals indexed in MEDLINE are now listed in searchable databases separate from MEDLINE. These require access to subscription CD-ROMs or subscription electronic search engines [e.g. ACP Journal Club, Clinical Evidence from BMJ Publishing Group, Cochrane Database of Systematic Reviews (CDSR), NHS Database of Reviews of Clinical Effectiveness (DARE), Cochrane Controlled Trials Registry (CCTR), Cochrane Review Methodological Database (CRMD), and Evidence-Based Medicine Reviews (EBMR) from Ovid Technologies] (see table 4). Many evidence-based clinical guidelines (another form of secondary overview) are also not listed in MEDLINE, but require separate searches of electronic guidelines databases such

Table 5. Hierarchy of evidence for individual clinical decisions regarding therapy

'N of 1' randomized trials
Meta-analysis of RCTs or 'mega-RCTs'[1]
Clinical standards from up-to-date guidelines produced by a cross-sectionally representative body generated according to systematic evidence-based methodology
RCTs
Clinical guidelines from up-to-date guidelines produced by a cross-sectionally representative body generated according to systematic evidence-based methodology
Systematic review of observational studies
Observational studies
Clinical options from up-to-date guidelines produced by a cross-sectionally representative body generated according to systematic evidence-based methodology
Physiologic studies
Unsystematic clinical observations

[1]Mega-RCT = Clinical trial with >1,000 patients as subjects.

as those maintained in the US (NGC), in Great Britain (NICE), and at other international sites (e.g. the Guidelines International Network) (see table 4).

The evaluation of the evidence gleaned from a proper search involves asking three questions: (1) are the results valid (i.e. a methodology and rigor of adherence to methodology assessment)?, (2) what are the results? (i.e. a precision, utility, as well as magnitude of effect assessment)?, and (3) will the results help me care for my patient? (i.e. a cost/benefit assessment, a local clinical care context assessment, and an individual patient appropriateness assessment) [22, 88, 89]. Many searches will lead to a plethora of clinical evidence, and many studies may come to conflicting conclusions. Obviously, not all conclusions can be correct. An EBM approach to sorting through the confusion involves the ranking of evidence from clinical studies according to the type of study design and the methodological rigor followed in each individual study as the first step. A proposed hierarchy of published clinical evidence for making individual clinical decisions is presented in table 5.

In general, there are five major sources of bias in clinical studies that could lead us to incorrect conclusions in applying those study results to our specific clinical decision: (1) selection of subjects to participate, (2) allocation of subjects between treatments, (3) assessment of treatment effect, (4) analysis of results, and (5) means of reporting the results. Uncontrolled trials are more likely to conclude that a treatment is effective and are more likely to overestimate the magnitude of a treatment's effect. As a result, controlled trials tend to be less biased than uncontrolled trials. Even among controlled trials, nonrandomized trials are more likely to conclude that a treatment is effective and are more likely to overestimate the magnitude of a treatment's effect [91]. The randomization process in RCTs theoretically should also take care of allocation biases that we have yet to think of or realize might be important. RCTs currently hold the pinnacle position for evidence hierarchy for these reasons.

Meta-analysis of RCTs and 'mega-RCTs' (trials with >1,000 subjects) hold a special place in the hierarchy because they include a clinical research subject size that maximizes statistical power, thus limiting the chance of a type 2 error (concluding that two therapies are the same or that a therapy is no better than placebo when, in fact, they differ by a small percentage in outcome probability). While meta-analysis of RCTs or a mega-RCT holds the pinnacle evidence position for clinical guideline considerations or healthcare policy decisions for a population, there is still an even more superior study for making a decision in an individual patient. This ultimate level of evidence for a clinical decision in an individual patient is a randomized, crossover 1 patient 'N of 1 trial' [92]. This type of trial eliminates all selection and allocation bias and the results, by definition, are always 100% applicable to your patient and their circumstances. The only bias that remains in this type of study for neurosurgery is the potential for placebo effect if the intervention(s) cannot be blinded to either the patient or the doctor. Unfortunately, a PubMed search July 11, 2004, for 'N of 1 trial' and 'neurosurgery' did not yield a single example of this type of trial published for our specialty (unpubl. data).

Whether or not the results of your search evaluation apply to your particular patient requires an analysis of the similarities and differences between your patient and those accepted for inclusion in the studies in question [62, 69, 73, 75, 88, 89, 93, 94]. In general, you should ask yourself if your patient is so different from those included in the study that its results cannot be applied to him or her.

Assuming your patient is not significantly different from the patients analyzed in the RCTs, the decision to apply those results in your particular circumstances requires additional analysis. It requires an assessment of: (1) whether or not the intervention or treatment is feasible or logistically possible in your circumstances, (2) a judgment regarding the likely magnitude of the probable effect of the intervention against the risk of harm, and (3) a full accounting of the patient's individual input regarding the impact of their own personal values, priorities, and desires on the choice before both of you. Formal clinical decision analyses are not suitable for this purpose because they use a group's strength of preference for different treatment options, which may not be applicable to an individual patient [95–97]. Again, the quality of the relevant evidence will impact upon setting your own threshold magnitude where the strength of effect will impress you and influence your decision making.

> 'Because of biases we describe in case-control studies, . . . you might not become impressed with their ROs [risk odds] until they reached 4 or more (some of our

colleagues would relax these guides for a serious adverse effect and set them even higher for a trivial one). Since cohort studies are less subject to bias, you might be impressed by RR [relative risks] of 3 or more in them. And because randomized trials are relatively free of bias, any RR whose confidence interval excludes unity is impressive and warrants further consideration' [98].

Objective statistics from clinical trials (e.g. odds ratios or risk odds and relative risks) can be converted into statistics that are more useful at the bedside and more intuitive for individual patient and physician decision making. These statistics include effect size (the difference in outcomes between intervention and control groups divided by the standard deviation), the number needed to treat (number of patients needed to treat to prevent one bad outcome), the number needed to harm (number of patients needed to be treated to produce one episode of harm), and likelihood ratios (for studies on diagnostic tests) [20, 88, 89].

Feasibility and logistical assessment include assessing whether or not the treatment in question is available in your setting. It does little good to conclude that a given patient with a ruptured aneurysms and subarachnoid hemorrhage would likely be better served by endovascular coiling of an unruptured aneurysm based on RCT data [96], if endovascular coiling is not available at your medical center and the patient is too unstable for safe transfer to another medical center that has the technology and expertise available. Likewise, it does little good to conclude that your patient with an inoperable single brain metastasis of suitable size should receive stereotactic radiosurgery in addition to whole brain radiotherapy for both length of life and quality of life benefits [97] if stereotactic radiosurgery is not available in your region. It also includes an honest and objective assessment of your likely results with an intervention compared with the success and morbidity rates of the surgeons published in the RCT. In one example, Swales [98] noted that the 'proven' advantage of surgery as a treatment for carotid stenosis was entirely negated by the 9.8% complication rate in community practice (study complication rate was 3.7%). In the absence of systematically acquired and analyzed objective data regarding your own outcomes for a particular intervention, one should at least take into account one's ongoing volume for the procedure in question. There are now many studies showing that surgeon case volume is clearly related to successful outcomes and lower complication rates for many neurosurgical diagnoses [99–107]. In the absence of the recommended technology, a significant personal ongoing case volume for infrequent or technically challenging procedures, or evidence that your personal outcome results are in line with those reported in the RCTs, one should consider referral of the patient if clinical safety concerns allow, and if the patient and family are agreeable.

As just stated, assessing the situation-specific probabilities of harm versus benefit for an intervention requires an objective knowledge and ongoing analysis of one's own success and morbidity and mortality rates for a given procedure. This component of evidence-based practice has been formalized by the AAMC, the ACGME, and the ABMS as 'practice-based learning and improvement', and is now one of the six 'core competencies' upon which we will all be assessed from now on. Without an ongoing objective and systematic analysis of your own results (usually through a prospective database), your perceptions, recollections, or estimations of your own clinical experience fall a level in the EBM hierarchy to the level of inadequately substantiated opinion. Practice-based learning and improvement fits neatly in EBM for individual clinical decisions, and indeed is a requisite for its proper application [84, 108].

Ultimately, clinical care of an individual patient requires multiple simultaneous and sequential decisions, and not every question that needs to be answered to guide those decisions can be answered with high quality evidence from the top of the hierarchy listed and ranked in table 5. A useful analogy here is one developed by Slawson and colleagues [109], which they refer to as a 'clinical jazz' approach. Just as a form of jazz music takes a defined piece of music (defined portions – evidence-based) and intersperses these defined segments with improvisational inspiration to create a beautiful, overall new, and individual creation. Clinical expertise and experience must fill in to provide guidance in equivocal situations between segments of the overall care plan which are firmly based on highest quality evidence.

It is also clear that certain aspects of decision making remain an art rather than a science. Even Straus and Sackett [94] admits that the 'optimal intelligible method of eliciting patients' preferences and providing decision support in a busy clinical setting is still to be determined'. This is particularly true for surgical interventions. In one landmark study, the attractiveness of surgery to patients was measurably greater when outcomes were framed in terms of probability of living rather than in terms of probability of dying, even when the figures simply reflected the inverse of one another [110].

Meta-Analysis Methodology

Meta-analysis of RCT's holds an important position in the hierarchy of evidence ranking of EVD (tables 5, 6). As a result, it deserves special focus and attention in any introduction to EBM and EBM methodology.

The educator and psychologist, Gene Glass and colleagues [111–113], introduced the concept and the term meta-analysis in 1976 as a means to quantitatively aggregate independent research studies. It was not originally described as a means of assessing RCTs. As clinical epidemiology has advanced, the original descriptions and methods have come to more closely resemble what are now referred to as systematic reviews, which include nonrandomized

Table 6. Clinical practice parameter evidence and recommendation ranking hierarchies

American Medical Association (AMA), 1990	US Preventive Service Task Force (PSTF), 1989	US Agency for Health Care Policy and Research (AHCPR, now the AHRQ), 1992
Class of evidence	Quality of evidence	Level of evidence
I. Prospective RCTs II. Studies where the data was collected prospectively and retrospective studies based on clearly reliable data (e.g. certain observational studies, cohort studies, prevalence studies, and case-control studies) III. Most studies with retrospectively collected data (e.g. clinical series, case reports, and expert opinion)	I. Evidence obtained from at least one properly designed RCT II-1. Evidence obtained from well-designed controlled trials without randomization II-2. Evidence obtained from well-designed cohort or case-control studies, preferably from more than one center or research group II-3. Evidence obtained from multiple time series with or without the intervention. Dramatic results in uncontrolled experiments (such as the results of the introduction of penicillin treatment in the late 1940s) could also be regarded as this type of evidence III. Opinions of respected authorities, based on clinical experience, descriptive studies, or reports of expert committees	I-A. Evidence obtained from meta-analysis of RCTs I-B. Evidence obtained from at least one RCT II-A. Evidence obtained from at least one well-designed controlled study without randomization II-B. Evidence obtained from at least one other type of well-designed quasiexperimental study III. Evidence obtained from well-designed nonexperimental descriptive studies, such as comparative studies, correlation studies, and case studies IV. Evidence obtained from expert committee reports or opinions or clinical experiences of respected authorities
Certainty of recommendation	Strength of recommendation	Grade of recommendation
Standard: Represent accepted principles of patient management that reflect *a high degree of clinical certainty* *Guideline*: Represent a particular strategy or range of management strategies that reflect a *moderate degree of clinical certainty*	A. There is good evidence to support the recommendation that the condition be considered in a periodic health examination B. There is fair evidence to support the recommendation that the condition be considered in a periodic health examination	A. Based on clinical studies of good quality and consistency addressing the specific recommendation and including at least one randomized trial B. Based on well-conducted clinical studies but without RCTs on the topic of the recommendation

Table 6. (continued)

Certainty of recommendation	Strength of recommendation	Grade of recommendation
Option: Remaining strategies for patient management for which there is *unclear clinical certainty*	C. There is poor evidence to support the recommendation that the condition be considered in a periodic health examination	C. Made despite the absence of directly applicable clinical studies of good quality
	D. There is fair evidence to support the recommendation that the condition be excluded from the periodic health examination	
	E. There is good evidence to support the recommendation that the condition be excluded from the periodic health examination	

observational studies, rather than modern meta-analyses. Unfortunately, authors sometimes use the terms 'systematic review' and 'meta-analysis' interchangeably [51] and there are no universally agreed-upon definitions of meta-analysis, per se [114]. Both systematic reviews and meta-analysis involve a systematic and quantitative review of smaller studies, ultimately yielding aggregate statistical results that take into account the statistically weighted contribution of each contributing study.

What is clear is that when most EBM practitioners refer to a meta-analysis, they are usually referring to a quantitative systematic review of RCTs [15, 51, 115–117]. Evidentiary-worthy meta-analyses employ a rigorous system for trial search and search quality control, rigorous criteria for selecting RCTs that share compatible selection criteria for inclusion, interventions and study endpoints, and rigorous statistical methodology for aggregating the results into the formation of a single new quantitative estimate of the effect of the interaction or risk factor. They also include formal analyses to assess for heterogeneity among included RCTs. Meta-analysis requires all the scientific rigor of an RCT. Detailed descriptions of methodology for meta-analysis of RCTs and for systematic reviews that include observational studies along with RCTs can now be found from multiple sources [51, 118–129]. Cumulative meta-analysis is a special form of meta-analysis that allows retrospective statistical definition of the minimum number of studies after which the question should have been considered closed [130]. Only a few meta-analyses of diagnostic testing [131–133], disease prevalence [133] and of RCTs currently exist for neurosurgery [134–142].

What is also clear is that a traditional review (e.g. 'case report and review of the literature', an expert review with selective reference citation, or a review of case reports and/or case series rather than clinical studies) is neither a systematic review nor a meta-analysis, as the terms are used in EBM. In order to be a systematic review or a meta-analysis, the literature search must be systematically inclusive and the inclusion selection judgments independently confirmed and verified. For secondary overview studies of therapies or interventions, the publications included must be actual studies that arrive at a quantitative effect statistic (e.g. an odds ratio for a case-control study or a relative risk for either a controlled observational study or an RCT). Traditional reviews result in more type 2 errors (failing to reject the null hypothesis) than systematic reviews or meta-analyses [143].

Clinical Practice Parameter Methodology

Clinical practice guidelines are defined as 'systematically developed statements to assist practitioner and patient decisions about appropriate healthcare for specific individual circumstances' [144]. An advantage of utilizing guidelines in clinical decision making over sole reliance on RCT results is that they take professional experience into account in an aggregate and more systematic manner, rather than on an individual or ad hoc basis [117]. Not only are more 'experts' involved in the consensus process (diluting out outliers in opinion) but in an evidence-based guideline development process, the opinions solicited are the experts' opinions about the collected evidence in the literature, rather than simply their own personal opinion regarding the subject.

Not all guidelines are equivalent in quality. The US NGC currently includes guidelines that have been formed through expert consensus alongside those based in systematic evidence-based methodology. It also includes guidelines that have been created by special interest and advocacy groups, subspecialty organizations, insurance companies, private consulting firms, cross-representative panels designed to include representatives from all potential stakeholders, and EPCs. Many of these guidelines conflict with one another, and there is currently no means of resolving or adjudicating these conflicts other than individual providers or oversight organizations making their own decision(s) as to which should take a position of supremacy or authority. The NHS approach to this problem is to only recognize guidelines produced by their National Collaborating Centers (table 2). These centers are each individually tasked with establishing representative panels, following validated guidelines methodology, surveying existing guidelines relevant to the topic and resolving any apparent conflict, and including both cost-effectiveness [39, 40, 90] and practicality as part of the final recommendation process.

According to Woolf [145], there are three main methods of guideline development – informal consensus, formal consensus, and evidence-linked development. From the standpoint of EBM, only the latter have evidentiary status for EBM decision making. Indeed, the US Institute of Medicine hopes to eventually restrict the use of the term 'guideline' to systematically developed advisory statements created according to validated methodology [144]. Some consider consensus guidelines as intellectually suspect by reflecting expert opinion, which when promulgated as a 'guideline' can formalize unsound practice [146]. Without strict adherence to systematic and validated methodology, panelists may be pooling ignorance as much as distilling wisdom [147]. Some guidelines are of questionable quality and there have been calls for guidelines on how to devise guidelines [148]. The use of guidelines is never a substitute for the exercise of professional judgment.

Construction of guidelines involves, first, a systematic means of identifying evidence and ranking the relative strengths, or quality of each study as evidence, and then, second, achieving panel agreement on a strength of recommendation linked to the analysis of the strength of evidence for each intervention in question. Both steps are critically important and have their own drawbacks and limitations. This two-step process evolved over several years in the late 1980s and early 1990s, with similar strategies taken by the US Preventive Services Task Force in 1989 [12], the AMA in 1990 [149–151], the US Agency for Health Care Policy and Research (now the AHRQ) in 1992 [13], and the Canadian Task Force on the Periodic Examination in 1994 [10, 11]. The hierarchical evidence rankings and strengths of recommendation for these schemas are outlined in table 6. It can be disconcerting to realize that the majority of neurosurgical practice ranks only Type C or an 'Option' recommendation.

The ultimate validity of any guideline is critically related to three key factors: (1) the composition of the guideline panel and its process, (2) the identification and synthesis of the evidence, and (3) method of guideline construction applied [152, 153]. The panel composition is crucial, both for ultimate acceptance of the guidelines by practicing physicians and for its critical influence on the recommendation step of guideline construction. Successful introduction of a guideline requires that all key disciplines contribute to its development to ensure ownership and support [154].

Panelists' recommendations can differ even when analyzing the same data. In general, studies have observed that US experts tend to be more action oriented than those from the UK, surgeons tend to be more certain about surgery than nonsurgeons, and generalists tend to be more conservative than specialists [147, 155–158]. Guidelines produced by advocacy groups and subspecialty societies tend to be most problematic and suspect, due to both problems with unbalanced panel representation and methodological concerns. There is a

Table 7. Criteria within scales classifying levels of evidence for clinical practice parameter development

Guidelines construction schema	Levels of evidence, n	Study design	Quality of study	Consistency of results
AMA [149]	3	X		
Canadian Task Force [10, 11]	4	X		
US PSTF [12]	5	X		
AHCPR (now AHRQ) [13]	5	X		
Guyatt et al. (EBM Working Group) [56]	6	X		X
Eccles et al. [167]	6	X		
Hadorn et al. [168]	7	X	X	
Ball et al. [173]	10	X	X	X
Liddle et al. [169]	5	X	X	X
Jovell and Navarro-Rubio [172]	9	X	X	X

natural tendency for advocacy groups to use evidence selectively for their cause [159]. Panels that overrepresent certain disciplines or exclude other key disciplines or dissenting voices may be seen as less credible [154]. Recommendations made by specialists sometimes are more influenced by the specialty to which they belong, rather than by the scientific evidence [160]. In addition, a recent survey of the methodological quality of guidelines produced by scientific societies indicates that even basic methodological principles are often being overlooked [161].

Ultimately, the quality and effectiveness of resultant guidelines depend at least as much on the quality of the consensus development involved in deciding the strength of recommendation (the second step of guidelines' construction), as on the quality of the evidence base [154]. Strength of recommendations is a complex topic that implies value judgments on top of methodological assessments of evidence. It should incorporate subjective considerations such as patient- or setting-specific applicability, trade-offs among risks, benefits, and costs [162]. Strong evidence for an intervention should not always translate into equally strong recommendations for use.

Detailed descriptions of methodology for constructing clinical practice parameters using systematic and validated evidence-based methodology can now be found from multiple sources [10–13, 27, 54–56, 149–151, 163–173]. As practice parameter construction methodologies have evolved, they have begun to take into account more than just the type of study design in assigning studies a level or strength of evidence score (table 7). Many methodologies now also include criteria for assessing the quality of the study [168, 169, 172, 173], as well as the consistency of results [56, 167, 172, 173]. Very few schemas currently take into account heterogeneity among studies [56].

As outlined in the section above entitled, 'The Role of Organized Medicine', organized neurosurgery has made efforts to construct clinical practice parameters based on evidence-based methodology [151]. The methodology chosen has been a modification of the original AMA approach [149–151]. Production of guidelines with a broadly representative panel based on systematic evidence methodology can take up to 3 years and cost hundreds of thousands of dollars [151].

The most successful and familiar effort to most neurosurgeons are the guidelines for the management of severe head injury [174], and the guidelines for the management of acute cervical spine and spinal cord injuries [175], from the Joint Section on Neurotrauma and Critical Care and the Joint Section on Disorders of the Spine and Peripheral Nerves, respectively. Additional joint section-sponsored guidelines include the guidelines for the acute medical management of severe traumatic brain injury in infants, children, and adolescents (Joint Section on Pediatric Neurosurgery and the Joint Section on Neurotrauma and Critical Care) [176] and the low grade glioma guidelines (Joint Section on Tumors) [177]. Additional section-driven evidence-based guidelines projects are reportedly continuing and slowly progressing across Joint Sections including initiatives focusing on penetrating cerebral injury, spinal fusion, glioblastoma multiforme, and cerebral metastases, among others.

Objections and Perceived Problems

EBM has not been embraced with open arms by everyone in medicine. Its degree of penetration across the country, within geographical regions, and among individual practices is highly variable at the present time, leading Sackett and Rosenberg [16] to remark, 'The future is already here; it just isn't evenly distributed yet.' However, I suspect that without the consistent support of, and investment in EBM by governmental agencies and organized medicine, it is not clear that its impact would have even penetrated to current levels. Many publications exist criticizing different aspects of the EBM approach [117, 154, 178–217], including a rather scathing editorial in 1995 from all the editors at a major medical journal [218]. Some of the criticisms are humorous [219] and some sound a somewhat bitter tone [193, 199, 201, 204, 205]. Even certain professional epidemiologists have some reservations [193, 206, 211]. The majority of critical articles have some kernel of truth to them and/or some constructive criticism. We will explore problems of style or perception in this section and more substantial limitations, problems, and constructive criticisms in the section that follows.

Disrespect and Conspiracy Theories

Unlike homeopathy, chiropractic, and early osteopathy efforts, allopathic medicine has always taken great pride in being strongly science-, and knowledge-based. Methodical evaluation and publication of clinical observations and experience were central to the Oslerian and Halstedtian traditions that flourished at Johns Hopkins and elsewhere in the late 1800s [220]. The landmark Flexner report [221] in 1910 transformed medical training by insisting on strong anchorage of medicine, and medical training, in the basic sciences. Rather than acknowledging a long and rich history of scientific approach to medicine, and presenting EBM as another stepwise improvement in a continually evolving process, many early advocates of EBM presented EBM as a revolutionary concept, or a radical 'paradigm shift' [15, 19]. Some in medicine felt that this approach was somewhat self-righteous, self-serving, and even disrespectful [218].

Many also felt EBM advocates were disingenuous in their approach, suggestive of a suspect underlying political or quasireligious agenda. The noted that early EBM advocates purposefully chose clever and highly emotive terminology that on the one hand, made EBM seem very desirable (what right thinking individual would not want to base medicine on evidence?), and on the other suggested that all that had gone before, as well as any people who disagreed with them, were not scientifically valid. If EBM exists, then non-EBM must also exist [180, 198, 199, 201, 204, 206, 210, 213, 218]!

Elitism and Arrogance

Regardless of the correctness and/or utility of the EBM approach, many have reacted negatively to what has been perceived to be an arrogant or academically elite tone in EBM publications [193, 199, 205]. Examples include published suggestions that the arguments of one legitimate critic were 'amusing', 'circular', 'good theatre', and of 'ephemeral interest' [222], or that practitioners who did not have the time to search and evaluate the primary literature themselves 'were at the mercy of the throw-away journals, drug "detailers" (pharmaceutical representatives), and traditional review articles' [88, p 13], or even published statements suggesting that doctors are more influenced by how many dinners were funded by the drug/technology company and how many consultancies they had had in making a choice than on the strength of evidence [24, discussion section, p 1212]. Some noted that leading EBM experts tend to be academic clinical epidemiologists who either no longer see patients as clinicians, or only see patients on an occasional academic sessional basis, who have allocated time in which to perform the multiple, time-consuming, and relatively complex steps of the EBM technique [117, 204, 205]. As physicians who may no longer be directly and personally responsible for individual patient outcomes (or only on an occasional basis), they run the risk of being out-of-touch with the realities of day-to-day clinical practice [117, 204, 205].

'Cookbook Medicine'

Some critics suggest that the EBM movement is an attempt to achieve a perceived ideal of standardized practice among doctors [198]. To many, this agenda seems most transparent in the clinical guidelines movement. In a worst case scenario, they foresee doctors reduced to performing 'cookbook medicine' involving technical application of clinical guidelines based largely on economic criteria [197]. The fact that the standards might be externally chosen and imposed, thus reducing physician autonomy, seems particularly ominous, onerous, and objectionable [187, 197].

Naiveté

Many point out that the practice of EBM decision making on a case-by-case basis can be very time consuming. They point out that most published EBM clinical scenarios used for illustration purposes are overly simplistic and usually only involve one formulated question for investigation [204]. Even for a single question, the assumption that there is usually one best way of doing things is an oversimplification of reality and may not be correct in many cases [213, 223]. EBM advocates may be naive in not recognizing the time constraints on modern clinical practice [214, 224] and not sufficiently acknowledging that clinical scenarios tend to be complex with multiple problems and questions in play at any given time [181, 191, 196, 204]. It is also pointed out that even if individual interventions have evidence to support their use, the more realistic scenario of using of multiple individual interventions in series, parallel, or a combination is not necessarily itself evidence-based, since the effects of interactions are unstudied [215]. To some EBM is merely an oversimplified attempt to convert healthcare into a series of technical problems to be solved through techniques derived using a narrow theoretical science approach. An approach which makes spurious claims of certainty in an uncertain world [197, 206]. Many would agree with Naylor [189] who stated, 'Clinical medicine seems to consist of a few things we know, a few things we think we know (but probably don't), and lots of things we don't know at all.'

Resistance to Change

It goes without saying that change can be unwelcome and resisted, particularly if the person perceiving pressure to change is happy and comfortable in the current state of affairs, if the change leads to time inefficiency and/or reduced income, if the change is perceived as reduction in autonomy, if the change requires retraining or education in new unfamiliar techniques and terminology, or if the change threatens their power base or self-image. Each of these is a potential negative perception regarding transition to EBM practice, depending on the individual concerned. Similar sources and levels of resistance accompanied the transition to a quality management or continuous performance improvement approach within health systems as embraced and endorsed by the Joint Commission on Accreditation of Healthcare Organizations (JCAHO) [225, 226].

At least some resistance may relate its potential impact on traditional medical and academic hierarchies where experience, rank, and seniority along with charisma usually are the route to being clothed in the mantle of 'expert'. In the traditional medical world, expertise remains in the realm of the expert, and esotericism is reinforced by exclusion of 'pretenders' from the discourse [187]. With EBM, the evidence carries the authority rather than the doctor. EBM levels the intellectual playing field in an academic department – everyone's clinical opinion counts equally regardless of rank or experience [224]. Knowledge based on a scientific discourse is democratic and open to debate, while knowledge based on expertise tends to be oligarchic and closed [187]. Tanenbaum [196] has gone so far as to remark that the EBM movement has sought to separate 'expertise from expert and knowledge from knower, and to locate the distillation of medical truth outside the clinical encounter'.

Substantive Problems and Limitations

The preceding section explored several objections to the expertise and authority, as well as style and approach of EBM advocates. Other objections centered around suspect motives of the EBM movement, the immaturity of a new concept still under development and evolution, and potential undesirable downstream implications of the movement. To some extent, these observations and concerns are objections to the messengers themselves or potential downstream effects of the message, rather than to the actual substance of the message. In this section, we look at substantive problems and limitations inherent within the EBM concept.

Lack of Proven Efficacy

Just like quality management and continuous quality improvement [226], EBM has been accepted and implemented without significant objective 'evidence' that it leads to improved clinical outcomes for individual patients or better health for populations [201, 204, 213, 216, 227]. In this respect, the ready acceptance and implementation of EBM by organized medicine and governmental agencies within the six competencies for medical education and maintenance of competency, and as the most legitimate basis for developing clinical practice parameters represent a huge investment based primarily on an unsubstantiated value judgment and hope.

That is not to say that EBM is entirely untested. In the 1980s, EBM was tested as a medical education strategy at McGill University in Canada in an

RCT. In the short-term, medical students taught EBM principles and techniques made better and more informed clinical decisions then their traditionally trained counterparts [5]. A follow-up study demonstrated that the EBM-trained group of physicians were better able to stay up-to-date and adjust their practice decisions to emerging clinical studies as long as 15 years after graduation [6]. Thus, while inefficient at rapidly building a baseline fund of core knowledge, it is a useful technique for identifying and evaluating new advances and discoveries, and clearly has a role in lifelong continuing education.

In respect to clinical outcomes, the impact of EBM has not been easy to assess [22]. The attempt by the NHS in Great Britain to produce an electronic journal to document this transformation (ImpAct published by Bandolier), only led to individual change stories and narratives, rather than studies of efficacy for EBC. The ImpAct experiment was apparently discontinued in 2001. While the impact of evidence-based practice parameter development on patient outcomes remains relatively understudied [228], there have been at least some suggestions of a beneficial impact. In a review by Grimshaw and Russell [152], only 17 of 91 studies on guidelines implications examined their subsequent impact on outcomes. Of those 17, 12 (70.6%) suggested a significant positive impact.

Literature as the Primary Source for Evidentiary Knowledge

A fundamental tenet of the EBM philosophy is that the peer-reviewed literature is the primary source or 'data mine' for identifying new clinical evidence. Unfortunately, neither the scientific peer-reviewed literature, nor our current means of accessing and searching this literature, are without certain limitations and drawbacks.

As Haynes [229] has pointed out, most scientific journals exist mainly to foster communication among researchers, and thus are a poor source of information for practicing clinicians. In addition, the journal manuscript review process is notoriously unreliable [230]. Even in the most reputable journals only about 10% of the papers will be original research or review articles that are ready for use [231]. Williamson et al. [232], in a review of reviews, estimated that only 6% of the literature published since 1970 is scientifically sound.

Probably the major systematic bias that exists in the scientific peer-review literature is publication bias. Publication bias has two forms. The first is the failure of negative or null studies to be submitted, or to be accepted for publication [118, 160, 233–242]. Studies with significant findings are inherently more important for building the reputation and promoting academic advancement of researchers (more likely to be submitted for publication), are inherently more interesting to journal editors (more likely to be accepted for publication), and are less likely to be blocked from publication under contractual authority by sponsoring corporations. The second form of publication is the tendency for the results of a single RCT to be published in multiple journals (duplicate publication), to be published at multiple periods of follow-up, or to be broken up for separate publication of multiple endpoints. Each of these latter situations can lead to 'double counting' in subsequent meta-analysis of RCTs or an individual EBM critical appraisal if this duplication is not recognized.

By definition, the peer-reviewed literature excludes books and book chapters. Yet book chapters can be an important source of clinical evidence in the form of RCT and other clinical study publication, as well as secondary evidentiary publications (e.g. quantitative systematic reviews, meta-analyses if RCTs, and cost-effective analyses). For neurosurgery, this takes on particular significance for systematic and quantitative analysis of surgical case series. For example, arguably the largest and most comprehensive microsurgical clinical experience, which has been systematically and quantitatively analyzed over a lifetime, has been that of M. Gazi Yasargil [243]. Professor Yasargil published this data in six remarkable books published over a period of 13 years [244–249]. When asked why he chose to communicate this information in book form rather than a series of journal articles, he replied that he had become increasingly frustrated with the unpredictability of acceptance of surgical case series articles in peer-review journals over time [Gazi Yasargil, pers. commun.].

Mining the literature data mine has become increasingly dependent on the MEDLINE database as well as electronic search software. Unfortunately, MEDLINE and related information technology databases are not comprehensive, not well indexed, and are not consistently indexed across time periods [192, 250]. Within MEDLINE, medical subject headings (MeSH headings) evolved and developed over time, and older segments of the database are not updated for cross-indexing with newer MeSH headings. New and established journals are continually being added to MEDLINE. MEDLINE only indexes journals back as far as 1966, but these early issues are only available for the first subset(s) of journals admitted to the database. While the database currently contains citations from more than 4,300 biomedical journals published in the US and in 70 foreign countries, journals from the US and Western Europe, as well as those published in English, tend to be differentially represented. It is also difficult for a clinician to look up possible therapies of which they are unaware.

As a result, relying solely on MEDLINE searches to identify clinical evidence can be problematic. Even restricting searches to RCTs, and relying on very thorough and systematic search strategies, MEDLINE searches have been shown to miss approximately one half of published trials [250–253].

Meta-Analysis

Meta-analysis holds a special place in the EBM evidentiary hierarchy, considered to hold greater statistical power and authority than all but 'mega'-individual

RCTs. Problems with meta-analysis stem both from imprecise or incorrect application of the term and from limitation of the procedure itself.

While advocates of EBM only place meta-analysis of RCTs ahead of evaluation of individual RCTs, the original definition of 'meta-analysis' (and that still subscribed to by many), also includes statistically analyzed quantitative systematic reviews that include observational, non-RCTs in this category [51, 111–114]. However, even a systematic review for therapeutic interventions is intended to be a review of clinical trials. It is clear that the term 'meta-analysis' was never intended as a fashionable replacement or descriptor term for a traditional review of case reports and small case series. Unfortunately, despite publication of several excellent meta-analyses of RCTs in the main American neurosurgery journals [134–142], our own journal reviewers and editors have compounded this confusion in our specialty by allowing nonclinical trial traditional reviews to be published, labeled or described as 'meta-analysis' [254–257].

Limitations of the meta-analysis methodology include difficulties with ensuring a thorough search for trials, ensuring reproducible and nonbiased trial selection procedures, and accounting for heterogeneity among trials included in the meta-analysis. Since MEDLINE searches only identify about one half of RCTs [250–253], careful searching outside of MEDLINE is a requisite. This includes, searching electronic databases of secondary systematic reviews, searching the pre-1996 peer-review literature, searching through known books on the topic and more general textbooks, searching the bibliographies of each identified trial, and searching for unpublished sources by searching clinic trial registries, reviewing abstracts from professional meetings, and personally contacting prominent researchers in the field. Unfortunately, while including unpublished RCTs reduces publication bias, it allows entry of trials that may suffer from poor methodological rigor, since they have not survived the peer-review process.

The reviewers themselves can also introduce significant secondary selection bias. This can occur as a result of failing to review the non-English literature, failing to have more than one reviewer and either having a biased strategy for including or excluding RCTs from the review, or leaving out an assessment of interobserver reproducibility for inclusion selection for the trial into the meta-analysis [258]. As a result, two or more meta-analysis done at the same time with the same access to the literature can reach different and even contradictory conclusions [259, 260].

Heterogeneity between the RCTs concerning inclusion criteria, samples, conditions, interventions, endpoints, or narrowness of focus are a major potential problem that can skew meta-analysis results [261, 262]. Heterogeneity among RCTs within a meta-analysis can be further compounded by the reviewing analyst who can intentionally, or unintentionally, scale or transform study results in ways that alter the apparent degree of heterogeneity [263]. Heterogeneity within a meta-analysis of RCTs is usually assessed graphically using a technique called a funnel plot [118, 241]. However, techniques such as funnel plots have been criticized for being chronically underpowered statistically [114].

These drawbacks and limitations inherent in meta-analysis methodology help explain why meta-analysis has occasionally led to results that conflicted with those of subsequent larger RCTs [258, 264–269]. A classic example is the lack of effect on mortality of Mg and nitrates in acute myocardial infarction despite promising meta-analysis predictions [270, 271].

Meta-analysis can also amplify the perceived impact of chance effects. Even if the odds of statistical significance from chance effect is <5% ($p < 0.05$), it is never zero for any given RCT. The classic example is homeopathy. A meta-analysis exists on 'good quality' RCTs showing that homeopathy might be of value for a wide range of conditions [272]. The problem is that any pharmacologic activity of an 'infinite dilution' is pathophysiologically impossible. Since a randomized trial of 'infinite dilutions' versus 'solution only' is a choice between two physiologic placebos, positive trials of homeopathy likely result from chance effects within individual RCTs, subsequently further amplified via meta-analysis [211].

The disagreement rate between subsequent large scale RCTs and previous meta-analysis of smaller RCTs is estimated to be 10–23% and is larger than one would expect from chance alone [258]. In one study of 40 outcomes in 12 subsequent large RCTs, the outcomes were not predicted by previous meta-analysis of smaller RCTs 35% of the time [268]. The positive predictive value of meta-analysis has been estimated to be only 50–60%, particularly if observational, non-RCTs are included in the 'systematic review' [273].

While attractive as a lower cost and efficient alternative to expensive and time-consuming mega-RCTs, meta-analysis clearly suffers from all the methodological drawbacks inherent in individual RCTs (see next section), and has potential to magnify those deficiencies to a degree that can lead to erroneous results. These drawbacks are disproportionately amplified if observational non-RCTs are included in the systematic review. Some have suggested that meta-analysis be downgraded to a weak tool whose main value is in the generation of hypotheses to be tested by specific mega-RCTs [203]. A more reasonable approach would be to recognize that meta-analysis with the intent of producing levels of evidence sufficient for evidentiary decisions (at either the individual decision or the guideline level) needs to be restricted to RCTs, and that it needs to be approached with all the thoroughness and rigor demanded of an RCT.

Inherent Limitations of Prospective RCTs

RCTs are extremely expensive and time consuming to perform [117]. The costs, logistical difficulties, and time required to complete enrollment, follow-up, and analysis are directly proportional to the number of patients enrolled, the expensiveness of the interventions and studies required to assess outcomes, and the length of time required to meaningfully assess the endpoint of interest. For new interventions compared against no therapy or placebo using standard statistical design, the number of patients needed in each study arm to demonstrate 5–50% improvements in an outcome endpoint per baseline incidence of that endpoint are given in table 8 [274]. Table 8 clearly illustrates that, unless the incidence of the outcome endpoint is very high in the control group, or the effect of the intervention is very dramatic in magnitude, the number of patients required can be daunting, or even prohibitive.

A simple perusal of table 8 will lead to the obvious conclusion that rare diagnoses and uncommon interventions are not likely to ever be studied using RCT methodology. As a result, there will never be this level of evidence for those diseases or interventions. Unfortunately, many neurosurgical diseases and interventions fall into this category. Additional reasons that RCTs may not be possible to perform include: (1) that a treatment has already been standardized at the institutional or third party payer level, (2) that the treatment may have already become regionalized beyond local influence, or (3) that the physician's or patient's perception of the treatment is too favorable compared with the alternative, to permit randomization [211].

Only interventions for conditions without preexisting effective therapies will have the luxury of being tested against placebo treatments or the natural history of the disease, and thus have the advantage for testing for larger treatment effects (e.g. 30–50% reductions in undesirable endpoints). Once standard of care (SOC) is established by RCT, alternative treatments for the same disease are usually tested against SOC rather than natural history or placebo. The truth is that there are often only small differences (e.g. 5–20%) in effectiveness between bona fide therapeutic options (i.e. those based on a coherent pathophysiologic rationale, those that have stood the test of time in accepted clinical practice, and those which have a basic science research foundation) [217]. As a result, clinical studies of additional or newer treatments are more likely to require mega-RCTs to demonstrate improved outcomes, or to result in null studies in smaller RCTs, and thus are less likely to be published or to be recognized as at least equivalent therapies (when in fact they may be superior). There is a clear advantage to being first.

RCTs also suffer from selection bias on the front end that can significantly call into question their external validity and generalizability for day-to-day clinical practice. The inclusion/exclusion criteria of RCTs lead to the selection of less complicated patients that may not reflect those seen in routine clinical practice [154, 182, 196, 199, 202, 203]. In some cases trials have included fewer than 10% of otherwise eligible patients [275]. In order for RCT results to be

Table 8. Numbers of patients needed in an RCT to demonstrate different reductions in incidence of a baseline outcome endpoint

50% reduction in endpoint				30–35% reduction in endpoint				11–20% reduction in endpoint				5–10% reduction in endpoint			
Ctl prop.	Rx prop.	per arm n	total n	Ctl prop.	Rx prop.	per arm n	total n	Ctl prop.	Rx prop.	per arm n	total n	Ctl prop.	Rx prop.	per arm n	total n
0.90	0.45	20	40	0.90	0.60	38	76	0.90	0.80	219	438	0.90	0.85	725	*1,450*
0.80	0.40	27	54	0.80	0.55	62	124	0.80	0.70	313	626	0.80	0.75	1,134	*2,268*
0.50	0.25	65	130	0.50	0.35	182	364	0.50	0.40	407	814	0.50	0.45	1,605	*3,210*
0.30	0.15	134	268	0.30	0.20	313	626	0.30	0.25	1,291	*2,582*	–	–	–	*
0.10	0.05	474	*948*	0.15	0.10	725	*1,450*	–	–	–	*	–	–	–	*

Italicized numbers indicate the need for a 'mega-RCT' with ≥1,000 patients.

Ctl = Control; prop. = proportion; Rx = treatment.

*Numbers listed assume a two-tail test for clinical significance, p set at 0.05 (5% risk of alpha, or type I, error), and 80% power (20% risk of beta, or type II, error) [274].

valid in the clinic setting for decision-making purposes, your patient must at least resemble the trial patients in terms of age, sex, pathological diagnosis, severity of disease, social class, dose and duration of treatment, concomitant ongoing diseases and treatments, and nursing care [276, 277].

In addition, RCTs often rely on measuring surrogate endpoints for outcomes rather than the actual outcome of greatest clinical interest. This may be because the surrogate endpoint comes about sooner than the endpoint it is supposed to predict (thus shortening the length of the RCT and reducing its cost), because it is easier to quantify, or because the surrogate outcome has a higher baseline incidence than the endpoint alternative, thus requiring fewer patients to demonstrate a significant change in a RCT (see table 8). Unfortunately, surrogate endpoints are secondary predictive outcome variables that can be misleading [203].

While selection bias still exists in RCT due to select population sampling for study, randomization is our best methodological means of reducing subsequent bias once the study is underway. Unfortunately, even randomization does not entirely eliminate bias during the treatment phase. Even in an RCT, it may be the case that a researcher's theoretical persuasion leads to their favorite therapy being administered in their study with more fidelity and enthusiasm than those to which it is compared [217]. Evidence for this assertion comes from two sources. First, studies of RCTs show that the treatment group ends up being repeatedly smaller, and statistically significantly smaller, than the placebo group by the time of analysis [278]. This suggests that patients are more often removed from the treatment group prior to analysis despite attempts at 'blinding' and 'intent to treat' modeling. Second, RCTs with outside sponsors more often report statistically significant advances than unaligned grant-supported studies [279].

Beyond considerations of practical feasibility, external validity, and residual bias within individual RCTs, lies an even greater concern. Namely, that by placing so much emphasis on the primacy of RCTs, EBM may be introducing a systematic bias into clinical decision making, guideline methodology, and healthcare policy decisions [199]. The effort and money required for RCTs is more likely to be spent on problems that are inherently interesting to clinical researchers and/or sponsoring corporations at the expense of less interesting alternatives that may be more important to our patients or the public as a whole [117, 185, 199, 280]. Pharmacological interventions will likely have an advantage over alternative treatments due to greater chance of corporate sponsorship, and easier introduction of patient and physician blinding compared with hands-on therapies or interventions [185, 211]. Ease and power of statistical analysis will favor easily quantifiable endpoints over equally important, but difficult to quantify endpoints, such as pain and quality of life [181, 185, 195, 196, 199,

209, 281]. Easier to measure endpoints will have an advantage over more difficult to measure (more expensive and/or time-consuming) endpoints [181, 185, 195, 209, 281]. Also, given the cost and effort involved, there is a tendency to study acute (rather than subacute or chronic) disease processes [185, 282], to study curative versus palliative interventions, and to measure short-term surrogate endpoints that may not always predict the more important longer-term outcomes of interest.

As a result there will always likely be a greater quantity of RCT evidence available in the literature for acute and/or fashionable disease processes treated with economically lucrative and/or fashionable interventions assessed using easily measured and quantifiable endpoints, than for chronic diseases, non-corporately-marketable interventions, or interventions assessed using difficult-to-quantify and/or measure endpoints. There will likely never be RCT evidence for sufficiently rare diseases, interventions, or procedures [184]. There will likely be more published evidence available for initially effective treatments (measured against placebo or natural history) than for subsequent potentially equivalent therapies (null studies compared with SOC). Relying on RCTs as best evidence of effectiveness can disadvantage older (often cheaper) treatments that have not been as rigorously evaluated as newer (often more expensive) treatments [154]. On the other hand, many newer interventions, particularly those in rapidly evolving fields or utilizing rapidly evolving technology (even if spectacularly effective), are unlikely to have been studied by RCT [192, 199].

Methodological Design and Rigor as Sole Arbiter for Levels of 'Evidence'

Methodological design is an important concern for assessing a clinical study in order to avoid the error of allowing bias to lead us to accept incorrect conclusions. Within EBM, RCTs are recognized as the methodology of choice to limit the misleading influence of bias. However, while excellent for studying therapeutic interventions, the RCT is a poor methodology for studying other epidemiological questions. Furthermore, there may be an inflection point where strength of effect should outweigh strength of methodology in assessing the level of evidence, or where the quality of a given study should lead it to carry more weight than a study of poor quality utilizing a less biased methodology.

RCT design is a poor methodology for answering or exploring epidemiological questions of potential disease etiology, pathophysiologic causality, therapeutic side effects, or describing new diseases [211]. Observational study designs are often the most informative methodology for exploring etiologic and pathophysiologic clinical research. The case-control study is the most potent research tool for studying side effects of interventions. Case series or even case reports remain superior for communicating new, unique or strange observations that may turn out to describe new diseases and/or lend insight into new treatment strategies or pathophysiologic understanding. RCTs tend to be most appropriate in remedial situations (when disease is already present) and less applicable in studying disease prevention (especially if baseline population is heterogeneous) [117]. Applying a methodologically based hierarchy for levels of evidence where RCTs remain at the apex in all these areas of medical inquiry may not be appropriate, unless the secondary analysis of the evidence (clinical decision and clinical practice parameter recommendation) adequately takes this into account.

There is a major difference between strength of effect for an intervention and strength of evidence supporting the use of that intervention [55]. Indeed there are interventions where the magnitude of effect is so strong with lower methodology analysis that the effect is very unlikely to be accountable by bias, and where failure to act on an individual case level or strongly recommend at a clinical practice parameter level is probably inappropriate. The introduction of penicillin in the 1930s and 1940s is a classic example. The dramatic effect of penicillin was obvious at the case report and case series levels. Whole inpatient infectious disease wards emptied as a result. It would not have been appropriate or desirable to await RCT testing before recommending penicillin as standard therapy for pneumonia. The introduction and application of nocturnal continuous positive airway pressure for hypersomnolence and sleep deprivation syndrome related to sleep apnea is another example [283, 284]. For neurosurgery, a good example is earliest possible, rather than delayed, intervention for patients with epidural hematoma and pupillary asymmetry [285, 286].

A hierarchy of levels of evidence based on methodology also fails to adequately account for rigor and quality within individual studies [206]. It is not at all clear that a poorly performed RCT deserves consideration as stronger evidence than a very thorough and well-done observational study. There may in fact be significant overlap between the categories such that the levels should be considered overlapping 'roofing shingles' rather than discrete and separate 'rungs on a ladder'. Mechanisms for adequately and consistently accounting for this issue are not yet in place.

From Guidelines to Polices and from EBM to EBC

At the public health and health management level, EBC is an attractive philosophy for providing an objective and science-based rationale for healthcare policies. Whether one is dealing with a formally nationalized health service such as Great Britain, or a US CMS service structured on a sustainable growth rate formula (where a relatively fixed amount of reimbursement money is allocated internally by shifting relative value units), we have entered an era of healthcare rationing. EBM has a potential role to play in making rationing less crude, arbitrary, and political [197]. Under this model funding can reflect guideline-driven priorities, and priority funding can be reserved for interventions with evidence of clinical effectiveness. Unfortunately, rationing implies cost-cutting and not just preferential funding, and EBM can be used as a cost-cutting tool [185, 201, 203].

The field of logic includes description of a classic logical fallacy where absence of evidence is interpreted as evidence of absence. This logical pitfall is particularly germane as a warning for attempts at EBC. Absence of proof of effectiveness of a healthcare intervention is very different from proof of lack of an effect [215, 287], and the presence of formal evidence for efficacy does not necessarily mean that this treatment option is superior to alternatives for which evidence (or evidence of an equivalent level) does not exist [185]. It is important to ensure that lack of evidence of effectiveness should lead to presentation of the treatment as an option rather than elimination of the treatment from funding or approval [164].

Much of accepted medical practice has never been validated in RCTs and there will always be plausible interventions for which no evidence is (yet) available [211, 288]. As a result, there will be large gaps or holes in any EBM clinical practice parameter effort attempting to codify clinical practice. Practitioners who limit themselves only to what is provable will preclude the use of many useful treatments [198], but it is not sufficient reason to withhold potentially beneficial intervention from patients [211].

RCTs tend to focus on quantitative and measurable endpoints. However, in healthcare not all that is measurable is of value, and not all that is of value can be measured [181, 198, 204]. Indeed it is a short step from a judgment that an intervention is 'without substantial evidence' to 'without substantial value' [181]. As a result, incorrectly interpreted or applied, some fear that EBM has the potential to devalue the unquantifiable in medicine [194, 198]. There is also a large difference between statistical significance and clinical significance, especially when the studied is evaluating a surrogate endpoint rather than the clinical endpoint directly relevant to clinical decision making and patient priority, or when the magnitude of effect is quite small despite statistical significance in an RCT [154]. Based on the systematic bias introduced by focus on RCT evidence discussed above, EBM could also bias healthcare and reimbursement policies against palliative care interventions, interventions for chronic diseases, therapies for rare diseases or uncommon therapeutic interventions, as well as non-corporately-marketable therapies (see section entitled 'Inherent Limitations of Prospective Randomized Clinical Trials').

Meta-analysis can also be misapplied with negative effects for funding and approval for health interventions. There have been several reports of the negative experience of having an incomplete or out-of-date meta-analysis, or meta-analyses performed by people without the subject matter expertise germane to the clinical condition in question, being adopted uncritically and effecting clinical decisions/policies [283, 289].

There is currently little strong evidence that guidelines substantially influence practice [117, 228, 290, 291]. Part of the reason may be that physicians tend not to think clinically algorithmically but rely more on pattern recognition as the most important part of differentiating problems [292, 293]. It may be that algorithmic protocols and guidelines are more suited to management planning than individual differential decision making [288]. Clinicians continue to rely on personal experience over research data. They tend to be realists rather than empiricists. Clinical trial evidence is considered only one of many forms of knowledge which can influence decision making. They tend to endorse and refer to guidelines most often for decisions that exist on the periphery of their experience [186]. Only when sufficient evidence has accumulated to challenge their original belief do physicians tend to alter what they believe [186].

In addition, not all medical questions are scientific in their nature, and many nonmedical factors effect decision making [204], including patient choice. Social or psychological components of the patient's problem may justify 'under'- or 'over'-management of the problem to achieve the individual goal of care [288]. Cultural differences in physician and patient beliefs, priorities, and expectations may need to be taken into account [294].

Even establishing EBM clinical practice parameters for every area of medicine will not likely, in-and-of-itself, be sufficient to transform healthcare into EBC. Assumptions that variation in healthcare is predominantly due to variations in approach of the physicians to the consultation rather than to effects of the environment surrounding the clinical consultation (e.g. economic constraints, resource shortages/limitations, regulatory constraints) are probably incorrect, or at least a significant oversimplification [203, 223]. Change must involve the environment of work and not just the individual physician [288]. Third party authorization limitations, economic constraints and counterproductive incentives may compete with the dictates of evidence.

Conclusions

Properly understood and employed, EBM is a tool of considerable value for medicine and neurosurgery. EBM is not a discipline onto itself within medicine [218] or a paradigm shift in the true Kuhnian sense [295]. Rather, it is a 'further developing and professionalizing the prevailing paradigm through a refinement of concepts that increasingly lessens their resemblance to their usual common-sense prototypes' [15, 19, 295]. It provides a secure base for clinical practice and practice improvement.

While less efficient than textbooks and didactic curricula as a means of rapidly acquiring a workable fund of clinical knowledge during medical and neurosurgical training, EBM critical appraisal training is an effective tool for keeping up-to-date with rapidly changing management strategies as part of lifelong learning and practice evolution. EBM is very effective for identifying gaps in clinical knowledge which can help us identify areas that need clinical research attention. However, as a closed, reductive, and deductive system, it tends to be relatively sterile for generating innovation, and for identifying potential strategies for filling these gaps. It is the soundest basis for developing and establishing clinical practice parameters.

With the support and backing of governmental agencies, professional medical societies, the AAMC, the ACGME, and the ABMS, EBM is likely here to stay. While some have argued that RCTs, meta-analysis, and guidelines have peaked in popularity, and are already on the decline [117], this is probably not correct. One can liken any perceived lull in penetration and impact to the time necessary for consolidation of an established beachhead, just prior to the definitive breakout and complete penetration across the countryside.

The fact that (1) EBM philosophy and critical appraisal techniques have become fully integrated into the training and culture of our younger colleagues (who will comprise an ever-increasing percentage of neurosurgical practitioners), (2) the fact that maintenance of certification will require individuals to demonstrate personal evidence-based practice based on tracking and critical analysis of personal practice outcomes as part of the performance-based learning and improvement competency, and (3) the fact that the progressively growing national healthcare expenditures (now approaching 20% of our gross national product) will necessitate increasing basis of reimbursement and funding based on evidence-based effectiveness and guidelines, all point to the likelihood that complete immersion of neurosurgical practice in EBM is inevitable. Widespread small-area variation in clinical practice and perceived high levels of avoidable error will also likely drive this effort. The EBM movement has convinced businessmen, politicians, bureaucrats and consumers that probabilistic knowledge of medical effectiveness is the means to better healthcare [196]. The fact that as of 2002, Wiebe and Demaerschalk [296] found most evidence-based care information sources substantially lacking in coverage of the neurosciences and therefore of limited use to clinicians in this field, simply reflects that neurosurgery has been relatively insulated to this point compared with other areas of medicine.

The transition to EBM within neurosurgery will not likely be easy or proceed without reluctance and resistance. Studies of innovation and change suggest that innovators pick things up regardless (~2.5% of the population), early adopters need written methods, scientific argument and credible sources (the majority preferring personal sources, opinion leaders, peer activities and reinforcement by social network), and late adopters usually require regulations, laws, incentives or sanctions, practical resources and provisions [297, 298]. Each of these latter possibilities likely lie on our horizon.

The healthcare policy implications of EBM and EBC are very real and deserve the careful attention of both individual neurosurgeons and our national organizations. Developing clinical accountability and a scientific rationale for rationing decisions and healthcare priorities is a rational managerial effort, but it will likely proceed at the expense of individual professional autonomy. Guidelines are important for advancing our field and the optimal care of our patients, but could become instruments of control. In differing circumstances of uncertainty, information (evidence) can be used for many purposes including ammunition in the struggle for influence to force or leverage decisions in favor of one stakeholder over others. It thus becomes critical that we continue to promote a strict and defensible evidence-based methodology for our own guidelines efforts, and that we keep pace with other medical professions and/or stakeholders who would establish 'guidelines' that might affect policies or healthcare decisions regarding neurosurgical diseases and interventions.

As outlined in this chapter, EBM is not without weaknesses and limitations, and the issues and controversies involved need to be understood by every practicing neurosurgeon. EBM finds answers to only those questions open to its techniques, and the best available evidence can be a far cry from scientific truth. EBM should not rob us of the ability to confidently function in a world of uncertainty that is inescapable in all branches of healthcare [184]. Yet knowing that the treatment prescribed is backed by solid evidence, and that we can proceed with clear a conscience, grants us a special form of freedom [203]. According to Naylor [189]:

> 'good clinical medicine must always blend the art of uncertainty with the science of probability' [but the] 'blend should be weighted heavily towards science, whenever and wherever sound evidence is brought to light'.

In surgery, expertise can never be fully separated from the expert. No literature review or number of RCTs or meta-analyses performed can ever make one an expert at clipping or coiling aneurysms, removing skull base tumors, or stabilizing a complicated spine deformity. In 1996, Sackett et al. [23] highlighted the importance of both evidence and clinical expertise, valuing the two equally:

> 'without clinical expertise, practice risks becoming tyrannized by evidence but without best available evidence, practice risks becoming rapidly out of date'.

Argument and counterargument by a mix of methodologic and biologic reasoning have always been the hallmark of medical progress [211]. To some extent this dichotomy reflects the old empiricist-rationalist debate [197], and within the tension between the two philosophies lies the fertile ground of innovation and new ideas. Clinical common sense is part of the art of medicine. By applying common sense along with empiric evidence, we effectively step outside the system to perceive a truth that is not apparent solely working deductively within a complex system [194, 207].

References

1 Cochrane AL: 1931–1971: a critical review, with particular reference to the medical profession; in Medicines for the Year 2000. London, Office of Health Economics, 1979, pp 2–12.
2 Chalmers I, Dickersin K, Chalmers TC: Getting to grips with Archie Cochrane's agenda. BMJ 1992;305:786–788.
3 Sackett DL, Haynes RB, Guyatt GH, Tugwell P: Clinical Epidemiology: a Basic Science for Clinical Medicine. Boston, Little, Brown, 1985.
4 Sackett DL, Haynes RB, Guyatt GH, Tugwell P: Clinical Epidemiology: a Basic Science for Clinical Medicine, ed 2. Boston, Little, Brown, 1991.
5 Bennett KJ, Sackett DI, Haynes RB, Neufeld VR, Tugwell P, Roberts R: A controlled trial of teaching critical appraisal of the clinical literature to medical students. JAMA 1987;257:2451–2454.
6 Shin JH, Haynes RB, Johnston ME: Effect of problem-based, self-directed undergraduate education on life-long learning. CMAJ 1993;148:969–976.
7 Brook RH, Davies-Avery A, Greenfield S, Harris LJ, Lelah T, Solomon NE, Ware JE Jr: Assessing the quality of medical care using outcome measures: an overview of the method. Med Care 1977;15(suppl):1–165.
8 Ellwood P: Shattuck lecture – outcomes management. A technology of patient experience. N Engl J Med 1988;318:1549–1556.
9 Harbaugh RE: Clinical outcomes analysis; in Linskey ME, Rutigliano MJ (eds): Quality and Cost in Neurological Surgery. Philadelphia, Lippincott William & Wilkins, 2001, pp 198–209.
10 Canadian Task Force on the Periodic Health Examination: The periodic health examination. CMAJ 1979;121:1193–1254.
11 Canadian Task Force on the Periodic Health Examination: The Canadian Guide to Clinical Preventive Health Care. Ottawa, Communication Group, 1994.
12 United States Preventive Services Task Force: Guide to Clinical Preventive Services. An Assessment of the Effectiveness of 169 Interventions. Baltimore, Williams & Wilkins, 1989.
13 Acute Pain Management Guideline Panel: Acute Pain Management: Operative or Medical Procedures and Trauma. Rockville, US Department of Health and Human Services, Public Health Service, Agency for Health Care Policy and Research, 1992, AHCPR publication 92-0032.
14 Guyatt GH: Evidence-based medicine. Ann Intern Med 1991;114(ACP J Club Suppl 2):A16.
15 Evidence-Based Medicine Working Group: Evidence-based medicine. A new approach to teaching the practice of medicine. JAMA 1992;268:2420–2425.
16 Sackett DL, Rosenberg WM: On the need for evidence-based medicine. Health Econ 1995;4:249–254.
17 Sackett DL, Rosenberg WM: On the need for evidence-based medicine. J Public Health Med 1995;17:330–334.
18 Sackett DL, Rosenberg WM: The need for evidence-based medicine. J R Soc Med 1995;88:620–624.
19 Crawley L: Evidence-based medicine: a new paradigm for the patient. JAMA 1993;269:1253.
20 Oxman AD, Sackett DL, Guyatt GH: Users' guides to the medical literature. I. How to get started. Evidence-Based Medicine Working Group. JAMA 1993;270:2093–2095.
21 Davidoff F, Haynes B, Sackett D, Smith R: Evidence based medicine. BMJ 1995;310:1085–1086.
22 Rosenberg W, Donald A: Evidence based medicine: an approach to clinical problem-solving. BMJ 1995;310:1122–1126.
23 Sackett DL, Rosenberg WM, Gray JA, Haynes RB, Richardson WS: Evidence based medicine: what it is and what it isn't. BMJ 1996;312:71–72.
24 Montori VM, Guyatt GH: What is evidence-based medicine and why should it be practiced? Respir Care 2001;46:1201–1214.

25 Meier B: Three senators seeking details for a drug-trial database. NY Times, July 9, 2004.
26 Omnibus Budget Reconciliation Act of 1989, Public Law 101-239.
27 Field MJ, Lohr KN; Committee on Clinical Practice Guidelines, Institute of Medicine: Guidelines for Clinical Practice. From Development to Use. Washington, National Academy Press, 1992.
28 White House Domestic Policy Council: The President's Health Security Plan. New York, Times Books, 1993.
29 Healthcare Research and Quality Act of 1999, Public Law 106-129.
30 Fletcher A: The NHS research and development programme and its impact on health care library and information resource centres. Health Libr Rev 1995;12:243–247.
31 National Health Service Executive: Priorities and Planning Guidance for the NHS: 1995–96. EL(94)55. Leeds, NHS Executive, 1994.
32 National Health Service Executive: Priorities and Planning Guidance for the NHS: 1996–97. Leeds, NHS Executive, 1995.
33 National Health Service Executive: Research and Development in the New NHS: Functions and Responsibilities. London, NHS, October 1994.
34 Scally G, Donaldson LJ: The NHS's 50 anniversary. Clinical governance and the drive for quality improvement in the new NHS in England. BMJ 1998;317:61–65.
35 Department of Health Press Release: Government keeps its promise for fairer, faster treatment for patients: the National Institute for Clinical Excellence opens for business. London, Media Centre, Department of Health, March 31, 1999.
36 National Institute for Clinical Excellence. Information about the work of NICE. http://www.nice.org.uk/page.aspx?o = 113677, accessed July 10, 2002.
37 Rawlins M: In pursuit of quality: the National Institute for Clinical Excellence. Lancet 1999;353:1079–1082.
38 National Institute for Clinical Excellence Press Release: NICE establishes guidelines advisory committee. London, NICE, NHS, May 23, 2000.
39 Rutigliano MJ: Cost effectiveness analysis: a review. Neurosurgery 1995;37:436–443.
40 Rutigliano MJ: Cost effectiveness analysis: theory, basis, and, methods; in Linskey ME, Rutigliano MJ (eds): Quality and Cost in Neurological Surgery. Philadelphia, Lippincott Williams & Wilkins, 2001, pp 285–294.
41 Stoelwinder JU: EBM in healthcare: management and policy. Med J Aust 2001;174:644–646.
42 Haynes RB: The origins and aspirations of ACP Journal Club. ACP J Club 1991;114:A18.
43 Haynes RB: So long, best evidence. Hello ACP Journal Club Online. ACP J Club 2001 (Nov–Dec);135:A13.
44 Guyatt GH, Rennie D: Users' guides to the medical literature. JAMA 1993;270:2096–2097.
45 Guyatt GH, Sackett DL, Cook DJ: Users' guides to the medical literature. II. How to use an article about therapy or prevention. A. Are the results of the study valid? JAMA 1993;270:2598–2601.
46 Guyatt GH, Sackett DL, Cook DJ: Users' guides to the medical literature. II. How to use an article about therapy or prevention. B. What were the results and will they help me in caring for my patients. JAMA 1994;271:59–63.
47 Jaeschke R, Guyatt G, Sackett DL: Users' guides to the medical literature. III. How to use an article about a diagnostic test. A. Are the results of the study valid? JAMA 1994;271:389–391.
48 Jaeschke R, Guyatt GH, Sackett DL: Users' guides to the medical literature. III. How to use an article about a diagnostic test. B. What are the results and will they help me in caring for my patients? JAMA 1994;271:703–707.
49 Levine M, Walter S, Lee H, Haines T, Holbrook A, Moyer V: Users' guides to the medical literature. IV. How to use an article about harm. Evidence-Based Medicine Working Group. JAMA 1994;271:1615–1619.
50 Laupacis A, Wells G, Richardson WS, Tugwell P: Users' guides to the medical literature. V. How to use an article about prognosis. Evidence-Based Medicine Working Group. JAMA 1994;272:234–237.
51 Oxman AD, Cook DJ, Guyatt GH: Users' guides to the medical literature. VI. How to use an overview. Evidence-Based Medicine Working Group. JAMA 1994;272:1367–1371.
52 Richardson WS, Detsky AS: Users' guides to the medical literature. VII. How to use a clinical decision analysis. A. Are the results of the study valid? Evidence-Based Medicine Working Group. JAMA 1995;273:1292–1295.

53 Richardson WS, Detsky AS: Users' guides to the medical literature. VII. How to use a clinical decision analysis. B. What are the results and will they help me in caring for my patients? Evidence-Based Medicine Working Group. JAMA 1995;273:1610–1613.
54 Hayward RSA, Wilson MC, Tunis SR, Bass EB, Guyatt G: Users' guides to the medical literature. VIII. How to use clinical practice guidelines. A. Are the recommendations valid. Evidence-Based Medicine Working Group. JAMA 1995;274:570–574.
55 Wilson MC, Hayward RS, Tunis SR, Bass EB, Guyatt G: Users' guides to the medical literature. VIII. How to use clinical practice guidelines. B. What are the recommendations and will they help you in caring for your patients? Evidence-Based Medicine Working Group. JAMA 1995;274:1630–1632.
56 Guyatt GH, Sackett DL, Sinclair JC, Hayward R, Cook DJ, Cook RJ: Users' guides to the medical literature. IX. A method for grading health care recommendations. Evidence-Based Medicine Working Group. JAMA 1995;274:1800–1804.
57 Naylor CD, Guyatt GH: Users' guides to the medical literature. X. How to use an article reporting variations in the outcomes of health services. The Evidence-Based Medicine Working Group. JAMA 1996;275:554–558.
58 Naylor CD, Guyatt GH: Users' guides to the medical literature. XI. How to use an article about a clinical utilization review. Evidence-Based Medicine Working Group. JAMA 1996;275:1435–1439.
59 Guyatt GH, Naylor CD, Juniper E, Heyland DK, Jaeschke R, Cook DJ: Users' guides to the medical literature. XII. How to use articles about health-related quality of life. Evidence-Based Medicine Working Group. JAMA 1997;277:1232–1237.
60 Drummond MF, Richardson WS, O'Brien BJ, Levine M, Heyland D: Users' guides to the medical literature. XIII. How to use an article on economic analysis of clinical practice. A. Are the results of the study valid? Evidence-Based Medicine Working Group. JAMA 1997;227:1552–1557.
61 O'Brien BJ, Heyland D, Richardson WS, Levine M, Drummond MF: Users' guides to the medical literature. XIII. How to use an article on economic analysis of clinical practice. B. What are the results and will they help me in caring for my patients? Evidence-Based Medicine Working Group. JAMA 1997;277:1802–1806.
62 Dans AL, Dans LF, Guyatt GH, Richardson S: Users' guides to the medical literature. XIV. How to decide on the applicability of clinical trial results to your patient. Evidence-Based Medicine Working Group. JAMA 1998;279:545–549.
63 Richardson WS, Wilson MC, Guyatt GH, Cook DJ, Nishikawa J: Users' guides to the medical literature. XV. How to use an article about disease probability for differential diagnosis. Evidence-Based Medicine Working Group. JAMA 1999;281:1214–1219.
64 Guyatt GH, Sinclair J, Cook DJ, Glasziou P: Users' guides to the medical literature. XVI. How to use a treatment recommendation. Evidence-Based Medicine Working Group and the Cochrane Applicability Methods Working Group. JAMA 1999;281:1836–1843.
65 Barratt A, Irwig L, Glasziou P, Cumming RG, Raffle A, Hicks N, Gray JA, Guyatt GH: Users' guides to the medical literature. XVII. How to use guidelines and recommendations about screening. Evidence-Based Medicine Working Group. JAMA 1999;281:2029–2034.
66 Randolph AG, Haynes RB, Wyatt JC, Cook DJ, Guyatt GH: Users' guides to the medical literature. XVIII. How to use an article evaluating the clinical impact of a computer-based clinical decision support system. JAMA 1999;282:67–74.
67 Bucher HC, Guyatt GH, Cook DJ, Holbrook A, McAlister FA: Users' guides to the medical literature. XIX. Applying clinical trial results. A. How to use an article measuring the effect of an intervention on surrogate end points. Evidence-Based Medicine Working Group. JAMA 1999;282:771–778.
68 McAlister FA, Laupacis A, Wells GA, Sackett DL: Users' guides to the medical literature. XIX. Applying clinical trial results. B. Guidelines for determining whether a drug is exerting (more than) a class effect. Evidence-Based Medicine Working Group. JAMA 1999;282:1371–1377.
69 McAlister FA, Straus SE, Guyatt GH, Haynes RB: Users' guides to the medical literature. XX. Integrating research evidence with the care of the individual patient. Evidence-Based Medicine Working Group. JAMA 2000;283:2829–2836.
70 Hunt DL, Jaeschke R, McKibbon KA: Users' guides to the medical literature. XXI. Using electronic health information resources in evidence-based practice. Evidence-Based Medicine Working Group. JAMA 2000;283:1875–1879.

71 McGinn TG, Guyatt GH, Wyer PC, Naylor CD, Stiell IG, Richardson WS: Users' guides to the medical literature. XXII. How to use articles about clinical decision rules. Evidence-Based Medicine Working Group. JAMA 2000;284:79–84.

72 Giacomini MK, Cook DJ: Users' guides to the medical literature. XXIII. Qualitative research in health care. A. Are the results of the study valid? Evidence-Based Medicine Working Group. JAMA 2000;284:357–362.

73 Giacomini MK, Cook DJ: Users' guides to the medical literature. XXIII. Qualitative research in health care. B. What are the results and how do they help me care for my patients? Evidence-Based Medicine Working Group. JAMA 2000;284:478–482.

74 Richardson WS, Wilson MC, Williams JW Jr, Moyer VA, Naylor CD: Users' guides to the medical literature. XXIV. How to use an article on the clinical manifestations of disease. Evidence-Based Medicine Working Group. JAMA 2000;284:869–875.

75 Guyatt GH, Haynes RB, Jaeschke RZ, Cook DJ, Green L, Naylor CD, Wilson MC, Richardson WS: Users' guides to the medical literature. XXV. Evidence-based medicine: principles for applying the users' guides to patient care. Evidence-Based Medicine Working Group. JAMA 2000;284: 1290–1296.

76 Guyatt G, Rennie D: Users' Guides to the Medical Literature: Manual for Evidence-Based Clinical Practice. Evidence-Based Medicine Working Group. Chicago, AMA Press, 2002.

77 Guyatt G, Rennie D: Users' Guides to the Medical Literature: Essentials of Evidence-Based Clinical Practice. Evidence-Based Medicine Working Group. Chicago, AMA Press, 2002.

78 Davidoff F, Case K, Fried PW: Evidence-based medicine: why all the fuss? Ann Intern Med 1995;122:727.

79 Haines A, Donald A: Getting Research Findings into Practice. London, British Medical Journal Publishing Group, 1998.

80 Florin RE: Outcomes measurement project started. AANS Bull 1997(fall);6/4:11.

81 Staff: AANS/CNS outcomes committee plans national pilot study on aneurysms. AANS Bull 1998(winter);7/1:7.

82 Harbaugh RE: Outcomes initiatives. AANS Bull 1999(spring);8/1:14–15.

83 Seaver MJ: Neuro-knowledge research partnership. AANS Bull 2003(spring);12/1:12–13.

84 Piepgras DG: Certification of neurosurgeons: a transition from neurosurgical certification and recertification to maintenance of certification. Report of the American Board of Neurological Surgeons. Clin Neurosurg 2003;99:1085–1088.

85 Gehlbach SH: Interpreting the Medical Literature: Practical Epidemiology for Clinicians, ed 2. New York, Macmillan, 1988.

86 Hulley SB, Cummings SR, Browner SW, Newman TB, Hearst N: Designing Clinical Research: An Epidemiologic Approach. Baltimore, Williams & Wilkins, 1988.

87 Riegelman RK, Hirsch RP: Studying a Study and Testing a Test: How to Read the Medical Literature, ed 2. Boston, Little Brown, 1989.

88 Sackett DL, Richardson WS, Rosenberg W, Haynes RB: Evidence Based Medicine: How to Practice and Teach EBM. New York, Churchill Livingstone, 1997.

89 Sackett DL, Straus SE, Richardson WS, Rosenberg W, Haynes RB: Evidence-Based Medicine: How to Practice and Teach EBM, ed 2. Edinburgh, Churchill Livingstone, 2000.

90 King JT Jr: Quantifying neurosurgical outcomes: how do we measure the effectiveness in cost-effective analysis?; in Linskey ME, Rutigliano MJ (eds): Quality and Cost in Neurological Surgery. Philadelphia, Lippincott Williams & Wilkins, 2001, pp 316–324.

91 Ioannidis JPA, Haidich AB, Pappa M, Pantazis N, Kokori SI, Tektonidou MG, Contopoulos-Ioannidis DG, Lau J: Comparison of evidence of treatment effects in randomized and nonrandomized studies. JAMA 2001;2286:821–830.

92 Guyatt G, Sackett D, Taylor DW, Chong J, Roberts R, Pugsley S: Determining optimal therapy-randomized trials in individual patients. N Engl J Med 1986;314:889–892.

93 Glasziou P, Guyatt GH, Dans AL, Dans LF, Straus S, Sackett DL: Applying the results of trials and systematic reviews to individual patients. ACP J Club 1998;129:A15–A16.

94 Straus SE, Sackett DL: Applying evidence to the individual patient. Ann Oncol 1999;10:29–32.

95 Llewellyn-Thomas HA: Investigating patients' preferences for different treatment options. Can J Nurs Res 1997;29:45–64.

96 Molyneux A, Kerr R, Stratton I, Sandercock P, Clark M, Shrimpton J, Holman R: International Subarachnoid Aneurysm Trial (ISAT) of neurosurgical clipping versus endovascular coiling in 2143 patients with ruptured intracranial aneurysms: a randomized trial. Lancet 2002;360: 1267–1274.
97 Andrews DW, Scott CB, Sperduto PW, Flanders AE, Gaspar LE, Schell MC, Werner-Wasik M, Demas W, Ryu J, Bahary JP, Souhami L, Rotman M, Mehta MP, Curran WJ Jr: Whole brain radiation therapy with or without stereotactic radiosurgery boost for patients with one to three brain metastases: phase III results of the RTOG 9508 randomised trial. Lancet 2004;363:1665–1672.
98 Swales J: The national health service and the science of evaluation: two anniversaries. Health Trends 1998;30:20–22.
99 Feasby TE, Quan H, Ghali WA: Hospital and surgeon determinants of carotid endarterectomy outcomes. Arch Neurol 2002;59:1877–1881.
100 Cowan JA Jr, Dimick JB, Leveque JC, Thompson BG, Upchurch GR Jr, Hoff JT: Impact of provider volume on mortality after intracranial tumor resection. Neurosurgery 2003;52:48–54.
101 Ruby ST, Robinson D, Lynch JT, Mark H: Outcome analysis of carotid endarterectomy in Connecticut: the impact of volume and specialty. Ann Vasc Surg 1996;10:22–26.
102 Barker FG 2nd, Amin-Hanjani S, Butler WE, Ogilvy CS, Carter BS: In-hospital mortality and morbidity after surgical treatment of unruptured intracranial aneurysms in the United States, 1996–2000: effect of hospital and surgeon volume. Neurosurgery 2003;52:995–1009.
103 Barker FG 2nd: Craniotomy for the resection of metastatic brain tumors in the U.S., 1988–2000: decreasing mortality and the effect of provider caseload. Cancer 2004;100:999–1007.
104 Hoh BL, Rabinov JD, Pryor JC, Carter BS, Barker FG 2nd: In-hospital morbidity and mortality after endovascular treatment of unruptured intracranial aneurysms in the United States, 1996–2000: effect of hospital and physician volume. Am J Neuroradiol 2003;24:1409–1420.
105 Kalkanis SN, Eskander EN, Carter BS, Barker FG 2nd: Microvascular decompression surgery in the United States, 1996 to 2000; mortality rates, morbidity rates, and the effects of hospital and surgeon volumes. Neurosurgery 2003;52:1251–1262.
106 Smith ER, Butler WE, Barker FG 2nd: Craniotomy for resection of pediatric brain tumors in the United States, 1988 to 2000: effects of provider caseloads and progressive centralization and specialization of care. Neurosurgery 2004;54:553–565.
107 Smith ER, Butler WE, Barker FG 2nd: In-hospital mortality rates after ventriculoperitoneal shunt procedures in the United States, 1998 to 2000: relation to hospital and surgeon volume of care. J Neurosurg 2004;100(suppl 2):90–97.
108 Manning PR: Practice-based learning and improvement: a dream that can become a reality. J Contin Educ Health Prof 2003;23(suppl 1):S6–9.
109 Shaughnessy AF, Slawson DC, Becker L: Clinical jazz: harmonizing clinical experience and evidence-based medicine. J Fam Pract 1998;47:425–428.
110 McNeil BJ, Pauker SG, Sox HC Jr, Tversky A: On the elicitation of preferences for alternative therapies. N Engl J Med 1982;306:1259–1262.
111 Glass GV: Primary, secondary, and meta-analysis of research. Educ Res 1976;5:3–8.
112 Glass G, Smith ML: Meta-analysis of research on class size and achievement. Educ Eval Policy Anal 1979;1:2–16.
113 Glass G, McGaw B, Smith ML: Meta-Analysis in Social Research. Beverly Hills, Sage, 1981.
114 Naylor CD: The case for failed meta-analyses. J Eval Clin Pract 1995;1:127–130.
115 Haines SJ, Walters BC: What is metanalysis? Surg Neurol 1994;41:381–388.
116 Chalmers I, Altman DG: Systematic Reviews. London, BMJ Publishing, 1995.
117 Maisonneuve H, Ojasoo T: From the life-cycles of clinical evidence to the learning curve of clinical experience. J Eval Clin Pract 1999;5:417–421.
118 Light RJ, Pillemer DB: Summing up: the Science of Reviewing Research. Cambridge, Harvard University Press, 1984.
119 Hedges LV, Olkin I: Statistical Methods for Meta-Analysis. Orlando, Academic Press, 1985.
120 L'Abbe KA, Detsky AS, O'Rourke K: Meta-analysis in clinical research. Ann Intern Med 1987;107:224–233.
121 Sacks HS, Berrier J, Reitman D, Anacona-Berk VA, Chalmers TC: Meta-analyses of randomized controlled trials. N Engl J Med 1987;316:450–455.

122 Hunter JE, Schmidt FL: Methods of Meta-Analysis: Correcting Error and Bias in Research Findings. Newbury Park, Sage, 1990.
123 Dickersin K, Berlin JA: Meta-analysis: state-of-the-science. Epidemiol Rev 1992;14:154–176.
124 Sackett DL, Oxman AD: The Cochrane Collaboration Handbook. Oxford, Cochrane Collaboration, 1994.
125 Clarke MF, Stewart LA: Systematic reviews of randomized controlled trials: the need for complete data. J Eval Clin Pract 1995;1:119–126.
126 Jones DR: Meta-analysis: weighing the evidence. Stat Med 1995;14:137–149.
127 Olkin I: Meta-analysis: reconciling the results of independent studies. Stat Med 1995;14:457–472.
128 Spitzer WO: The Potsdam International Consultation on Meta-Analysis. J Clin Epidemiol 1995;48:1–171.
129 Cook DJ, Sackett DL, Spitzer WO: Methodologic guidelines for systematic reviews of randomized controlled trials in health care from the Potsdam Consultation on Meta-Analysis. J Clin Epidemiol 1995;48:167–171.
130 Lau J, Antman EM, Jimenez-Silva J, Kupelnick B, Mosteller F, Chalmers TC: Cumulative meta-analysis of therapeutic trials for myocardial infarction. N Engl J Med 1992;327:248–254.
131 Hofman PAM, Nelemans P, Kemerink, GJ, Wilmink JT: Value of radiological diagnosis of skull fracture in the management of mild head injury: meta-analysis. J Neurol Neurosurg Psychiatry 2000;68:416–422.
132 Chappell ET, Moure FC, Good MC: Comparison of computed tomographic angiography with digital subtraction angiography in the diagnosis of cerebral aneurysms: a meta-analysis. Neurosurgery 2003;52:624–631.
133 Cloft HJ, Kallmes DF, Kallmes MH, Goldstein JH, Jensen ME, Dion JE: Prevalence of cerebral aneurysms in patients with fibromuscular dysplasia: a reassessment. J Neurosurg 1998;88:436–440.
134 Langley JM, LeBlanc JC, Drake J, Milner R: Efficacy of antimicrobial prophylaxis in placement of cerebrospinal fluid shunts: meta-analysis. Clin Infect Dis 1993;17:98–103.
135 Barker FG 2nd: Efficacy of prophylactic antibiotics for craniotomy: a meta-analysis. Neurosurgery 1994;35:484–492.
136 Di Mascio R, Marchioli R, Tognoni G: From pharmacological promises to controlled clinical trials to meta-analysis and back: the case of nimodipine in cerebrovascular disorders. Clin Trials Metaanal 1994;29:57–79.
137 Haines SJ, Walters BC: Antibiotic prophylaxis for cerebrospinal fluid shunts: a metanalysis. Neurosurgery 1994;34:87–92.
138 Barker FG 2nd, Ogilvy CS: Efficacy of prophylactic nimodipine for delayed ischemic deficit after subarachnoid hemorrhage: a meta-analysis. J Neurosurg 1996;84:405–414.
139 Barker FG 2nd: Efficacy of prophylactic antibiotics in cerebrospinal shunt surgery: a meta-analysis. Neurosurgery 1998;43:694.
140 Prabhu VC, Kaufman HH, Voelker JL, Aronoff SC, Niewiadomska-Bugaj M, Mascaro S, Hobbs GR: Prophylactic antibiotics with intracranial pressure monitors and external ventricular drains: a review of the evidence. Surg Neurol 1999;52:226–237.
141 Farace E, Alves W: Do women fare worse: a metaanalysis of gender differences in traumatic brain injury outcome. J Neurosurg 2000;93:539–545.
142 Barker FG 2nd: Efficacy of prophylactic antibiotic therapy in spinal surgery: a meta-analysis. Neurosurgery 2002;51:391–401.
143 Cooper HM, Rosenthal R: Statistical versus traditional procedures for summarizing research findings. Psychol Bull 1980;87:442–449.
144 Field MJ, Lohr KN, Institute of Medicine, Committee to Advise the Public Health Service on Clinical Practice Guidelines: Clinical Practice Guidelines: Directions for a New Program. Washington, National Academy Press, 1990.
145 Woolf SH: Practice guidelines, a new reality in medicine. II. Methods of developing guidelines. Arch Intern Med 1992;152:946–952.
146 Delamothe T: Wanted: guidelines that doctors will follow. Implementation is the problem. BMJ 1993;307:218.
147 Scott EA, Black N: When does consensus exist in expert panels? J Public Health Med 1991;13:35–39.

148 Jackson R, Feder G: Guidelines for clinical guidelines: a simple, pragmatic strategy for guideline development. BMJ 1998;317:427–428.
149 AMA: Office of Quality Insurance and Healthcare Organizations' Attributes to Guideline Development of Practice Parameters. Chicago, AMA, 1990.
150 Rosenberg J, Greenberg MK: Practice parameters: strategies for survival into the nineties. Neurology 1992;42:1110–1115.
151 Walters BC: Clinical practice parameter development in neurosurgery; in Bean JR (ed): Neurosurgery in Transition: The Socioeconomic Transformation of Neurological Surgery. Baltimore, Williams & Wilkins, 1998, pp 99–111.
152 Grimshaw JM, Russell IT: Effect of clinical guidelines on medical practice: a systematic review of rigorous evaluations. Lancet 1993;342:1317–1322.
153 Grimshaw J, Russell I: Achieving health gain through clinical guidelines. I. Developing scientifically valid guidelines. Qual Health Care 1993;2:243–248.
154 Grimshaw J, Eccles M, Russell I: Developing clinically valid practice guidelines. J Eval Clin Pract 1995;1:37–48.
155 Brook RH, Kosecoff JB, Park RE, Chassin MR, Winslow CM, Hampton JR: Diagnosis and treatment of coronary disease: comparison of doctors' attitudes in the USA and the UK. Lancet 1988;i:750–753.
156 Kahn KL, Park RE, Brook RH, Chassin MR, Kosecoff J, Fink A, Keesey JW, Solomon DH: The effect of comorbidity on appropriateness ratings for two gastrointestinal procedures. J Clin Epidemiol 1988;41:115–122.
157 Leape LL, Park RE, Kahan JP, Brook RH: Group judgments of appropriateness: the effect of panel composition. Qual Assur Health Care 1992;4:151–159.
158 Fraser GM, Pilpel D, Hollis S, Kosecoff J, Brook RH: Indications for cholecystectomy: the results of a consensus panel approach. Qual Assur Health Care 1993;5:75–80.
159 Larson EB: Evidence-based medicine: is translating evidence into practice a solution to the cost-quality challenges facing medicine? Jt Comm J Qual Improv 1999;25:480–485.
160 Chalmers TC, Frank CS, Reitman D: Minimizing the three stages of publication bias. JAMA 1990;263:1392–1395.
161 Shaneyfelt TM, Mayo-Smith MF, Rothwangl J: Are guidelines following guidelines? The methodological quality of clinical practice guidelines in the peer-reviewed medical literature. JAMA 1999;281:1950–1951.
162 Liberati A, Buzzetti R, Grilli R, Magrini N, Minozzi S: Which guidelines can we trust? Assessing strength of evidence behind recommendations for clinical practice. West J Med 2001;174: 262–265.
163 Woolf SH, Battista R, Anderson GM, Logan AG, Wang E: Assessing the clinical effectiveness of preventive maneuvers: analytic principles and systematic methods in reviewing evidence and developing clinical practice recommendations. A report by the Canadian Task Force on the Periodic Health Examination. J Clin Epidemiol 1990;43:891–905.
164 Eddy DM: A Manual for Assessing Health Practices and Designing Practice Policies: the Explicit Approach. Philadelphia, American College of Physicians, 1992.
165 United States Congress, Office of Technology Assessment: Identifying Health Technologies That Work. Searching for Evidence. Washington, United States Government Printing Office, 1994, publication No OTA-H-608.
166 Field MJ, Institute of Medicine, Committee on Methods for Setting Priorities for Guidelines Development, Division of Health Care Services: Setting Priorities for Clinical Practice Guidelines. Washington, National Academy Press, 1995.
167 Eccles M, Clapp Z, Grimshaw J, Adams PC, Higgins B, Purves I, Russell I: North of England evidence based guidelines development project: methods of guideline development. BMJ 1996;312:760–762.
168 Hadorn DC, Baker D, Hodges JS, Hicks N: Rating the quality of evidence for clinical practice guidelines. J Clin Epidemiol 1996;49:749–754.
169 Liddle J, Williams M, Irwig L: Method for evaluating research and guideline evidence. Sydney, New South Wales Health Department, 1996. http://www.health.nsw.gov.au/public-health/crcp/publications/general/merge.html

170 United States Preventive Services Task Force: Guide to Clinical Preventive Services, ed 2. Baltimore, Williams & Wilkins, 1996.
171 Woolf SH, DiGuiseppi CG, Atkins D, Kamerow DB: Developing evidence-based clinical practice guidelines: lessons learned by the US Preventive Services Task Force. Annu Rev Public Health 1996;17:511–538.
172 Jovell AL, Navarro-Rubio MD: Evaluacion de la evidencia cientifica. Med Clin (Barc) 1997;105: 740–743.
173 Ball C, Phillips B, Sackett D, Badenoch D, Straus S, Haynes B, Dawes M: Levels of Evidence and Grades of Recommendation. Oxford, Oxford Centre for Evidence-Based Medicine, 1998. http://www.cebm.net/levels_of_evidence.asp
174 Brain Trauma Foundation. Guidelines for severe head injury management. J Neurotrauma 1996;13:639–731.
175 Section on Disorders of the Spine and Peripheral Nerves: Guidelines for the management of acute cervical spine and spinal cord injuries. Neurosurgery 2002;50(suppl 3):1–199.
176 Adelson PD, et al., American Association for Surgery of Trauma: Guidelines for the acute medical management of severe traumatic brain injury in infants, children, and adolescents. Pediatr Crit Care Med 2003;4(suppl 3):S1–S75.
177 Low Grade Glioma Guidelines Team: Practice parameters in adults with suspected or known supratentorial nonoptic pathway low-grade glioma. Neurosurg Focus 1998;4:article 10.
178 Tanenbaum SJ: What physicians know. N Engl J Med 1993;329:1268–1271.
179 Tanenbaum SJ: Knowing and acting in medical practice: the epistemological politics of outcomes research. J Health Polit Policy Law 1994;19:27–44.
180 Blau JN: Evidence-based medicine. Lancet 1995;346:1300.
181 Bradley F, Field J: Evidence-based medicine. Lancet 1995;346:838–839.
182 Charlton BG: Evidence based medicine: megatrials are subordinate to medical science. BMJ 1995;311:257.
183 Clarke MJ, Stewart LA: Systematic reviews of randomized controlled trials: the need for complete data. J Eval Clin Pract 1995;1:119–126.
184 Jones GW, Sagar SM: Evidence based medicine. No guidance is provided for situations for which evidence is lacking. BMJ 1995;311:258.
185 Hope T: Evidence based medicine and ethics. J Med Ethics 1995;21:259–260.
186 Hunter DJ: Effective practice. J Eval Clin Pract 1995;1:131–134.
187 Marshall T: Evidence-based medicine. Lancet 1995;346:1171–1172.
188 Naylor CD: The case for failed meta-analyses. J Eval Clin Pract 1995;1:127–130.
189 Naylor CD: Grey zones of clinical practice: some limits to evidence-based medicine. Lancet 1995;345:840–842.
190 Norman G: Evidence-based medicine. Lancet 1995;346:1300.
191 O'Rourke MF: The move towards evidence-based medicine. Med J Aust 1995;163:332–333.
192 Rigge M: Consumer audit. A speech to the second National Medical and Dental Audit Conference, 4 April 1995. J Eval Clin Pract 1995;1:135–140.
193 Shahar E: Evidence-based medicine. Lancet 1995;346:1172.
194 Sleigh JW: Evidence-based medicine and Kurt Godel. Lancet 1995;346:1172.
195 Smith BH: Evidence-based medicine: quality cannot always be quantified. BMJ 1995;311:258.
196 Tanenbaum S: Getting there from here: evidentiary quandaries of the US outcomes movement. J Eval Clin Pract 1995;1:97–103.
197 Hunter DJ: Rationing and evidence-based medicine. J Eval Clin Pract 1996;2:5–8.
198 Polychronis A, Miles A, Bentley P: Evidence-based medicine: reference? Dogma? Neologism? New orthodoxy? J Eval Clin Pract 1996;2:1–3.
199 Polychronis A, Miles A, Bentley P: The protagonists of 'evidence-based medicine': arrogant, seductive and controversial. J Eval Clin Pract 1996;2:9–12.
200 Blau JN: Evidence-based medicine. J Eval Clin Pract 1997;3:149–151.
201 Charlton BG: Restoring the balance: evidence-based medicine put in its place. J Eval Clin Pract 1997;3:87–98.
202 Feinstein AR, Horwitz RI: Problems in the 'evidence' of 'evidence-based medicine'. Am J Med 1997;103:529–535.

203 Hampton JR: Evidence-based medicine, practice variations and clinical freedom. J Eval Clin Pract 1997;3:123–131.
204 Miles A, Bentley P, Polychronis A, Grey J: Evidence-based medicine: why all the fuss? This is why. J Eval Clin Pract 1997;3:83–86.
205 Morgan WKC: On evidence, embellishment and efficacy. J Eval Clin Pract 1997;3:117–122.
206 Shahar E: A Popperian perspective of the term 'evidence-based medicine'. J Eval Clin Pract 1997;3:109–116.
207 Sleigh JW: Logical limits of randomized controlled trials. J Eval Clin Pract 1997;3:145–148.
208 Black D: The limitations of evidence. J R Coll Physicians Lond 1998;32:23–26.
209 Kerridge I, Lowe M, Henry D: Ethics and evidence based medicine. BMJ 1998;316:1151–1153.
210 Tonelli MR: The philosophical limits of evidence-based medicine. Acad Med 1998;73: 1234–1240.
211 Vandenbroucke JP: Observational research and evidence-based medicine: what should we teach young physicians? J Clin Epidemiol 1998;51:467–472.
212 Clarke JB: Evidence-based practice: a retrograde step? The importance of pluralism in evidence generation for the practice of health care. J Clin Nurs 1999;8:89–94.
213 Goodman NW: Who will challenge evidence-based medicine? J R Coll Physicians Lond 1999;33:249–251.
214 Lalwani SI, Olive DL: Problems with evidence-based medicine. J Am Assoc Gynecol Laparosc 1999;6:237–240.
215 Van Weel C, Knottnerus JA: Evidence-based interventions and comprehensive treatment. Lancet 1999;353:916–918.
216 Goodman NW: In my view . . . Criticizing evidence-based medicine. Thyroid 2000;10:157–160.
217 Messer SB: Empirically supported treatments: cautionary notes. Medscape Gen Med 2002;4:13. http://www.medscape.com/viewarticle/445082.
218 Editorial: Evidence-based medicine, in its place. Lancet 1995;346:785.
219 Grahame-Smith D: Evidence based medicine: Socratic dissent. BMJ 1995;310:1126–1127.
220 Osler W: The Principles and Practice of Medicine: Designed for the Use of Practitioners and Students of Medicine. New York, Appleton, 1982.
221 Flexner A: Medical Education in the United States and Canada: a Report to the Carnegie Foundation for the Advancement of Teaching. New York, Merrymount Press, 1910.
222 Sackett D: Evidence-based medicine. Lancet 1995;346:1171–1172.
223 Aveyard P: Evidence-based medicine and public health. J Eval Clin Pract 1997;3:139–144.
224 Grimes DA: Introducing evidence-based medicine into a department of obstetrics and gynecology. Obstet Gynecol 1995;86:451–457.
225 Linskey ME: The total quality movement: a paradigm shift in leadership and management philosophy for neurological surgery and health care in general; in Linskey ME, Rutigliano MJ (eds): Quality and Cost in Neurological Surgery. Philadelphia, Lippincott Williams & Wilkins, 2001, pp 3–31.
226 Linskey ME: Obstacles to implementing a quality philosophy in neurological surgery; in Linskey ME, Rutigliano MJ (eds): Quality and Cost in Neurological Surgery. Philadelphia, Lippincott Williams & Wilkins, 2001, pp 260–284.
227 Leung GM: Evidence-based practice revisited. Asia Pac J Public Health 2001;13:116–121.
228 Grol R: Between evidence-based practice and total quality management: the implementation of cost-effective care. Int J Qual Health Care 2000;12:297–304.
229 Haynes RB: Loose connections between peer-reviewed clinical journals and clinical practice. Ann Intern Med 1990;113:724–728.
230 Whitehurst GJ: Interrater agreement for journal manuscript reviews. Am Psychol 1984;39:22–28.
231 Haynes RB, Sackett DL, Gray JAM, Cook DL, Guyatt GH: Transferring evidence from research into practice. 2. Getting the evidence straight. Evid Based Med 1997;2:4–6.
232 Williamson JW, Goldschmidt PG, Colton T: The quality of medical literature: an analysis of validation assessments; in Bailar JC 3rd, Mosteller F (eds): Medical Uses of Statistics. Waltham, NEJM Books, 1986, pp 370–391.
233 Rosenthal R: The file drawer problem and tolerance for null results. Psychol Bull 1979;86: 638–641.

234 Begg CB, Berlin JA: Publication bias: a problem in interpreting medical data. J R Stat Soc 1988;151:419–463.
235 Dickersin K, Chan S, Chalmers TC, Sacks HS, Smith H Jr: Publication bias and clinical trials. Control Clin Trials 1987;8:343–353.
236 Dickersin K: The existence of publication bias and risk factors for its occurrence. JAMA 1990;263:1385–1389.
237 Easterbrook PJ, Berlin JA, Gopalan R, Matthews DR: Publication bias in clinical research. Lancet 1991;337:867–872.
238 Dickersin K, Min YI, Meinert CL: Factors influencing publication of research results. Follow-up of applications submitted to two institutional review boards. JAMA 1992;267:374–378.
239 Dickersin K, Min YI: NIH clinical trials and publication bias. Online J Curr Clin Trials 1993;Doc No 50.
240 Dickersin K, Min YI: Publication bias: the problem that won't go away. Ann NY Acad Sci 1993;703:135–146.
241 Egger M, Davey-Smith G, Schneider M, Minder C: Bias in meta-analysis detected by a simple, graphical test. BMJ 1997;315:629–634.
242 Sterne JA, Egger M, Smith GD: Systematic reviews in health care: investigating and dealing with publication and other biases in meta-analysis. BMJ 2001;323:101–105.
243 Apuzzo MLJ: Legacies. Man of the century 1950–1999, M Gazi Yasargil (series of 4 articles). Neurosurgery 1999;45:1010–1092.
244 Yasargil MG: Microneurosurgery. New York, Thieme, 1984, vol 1.
245 Yasargil MG: Microneurosurgery. New York, Thieme, 1984, vol 2.
246 Yasargil MG: Microneurosurgery. New York, Thieme, 1987, vol 3A.
247 Yasargil MG: Microneurosurgery. New York, Thiemeg, 1988, vol 3B.
248 Yasargil MG: Microneurosurgery. New York, Thieme, 1994, vol 4A.
249 Yasargil MG: Microneurosurgery. New York, Thieme, 1996, vol 4B.
250 Dickersin K, Scherer R, Lefebvre C: Identifying relevant studies for systematic reviews. BMJ 1994;309:1286–1291.
251 Bernstein F: The retrieval of randomized clinical trials in liver diseases from the medical literature: manual versus MEDLARS searches. Control Clin Trials 1988;9:23–31.
252 Dickersin K, Hewitt P, Mutch L, Chalmers I, Chalmers TC: Perusing the literature: comparison of MEDLINE searching with a perinatal trials database. Control Clin Trials 1985;6:306–317.
253 Poynard T, Conn HO: The retrieval of randomized clinical trials in liver disease from the medical literature. A comparison of MEDLARS and manual methods. Control Clin Trials 1985;6: 271–279.
254 Awad IA, Little JR, Akarawi WP, Ahl J: Intracranial dural arteriovenous malformations: factors predisposing to an aggressive neurological course. J Neurosurg 1990;72:839–850.
255 Canavero S, Pagni CA, Duca S, Bradac GB: Spinal intramedullary cavernous angiomas: a literature metaanalysis. Surg Neurol 1994;41:381–388.
256 King JT Jr, Berlin JA, Flamm ES: Morbidity and mortality from elective surgery for asymptomatic, unruptured, intracranial aneurysms: a meta-analysis. J Neurosurg 1994;81:837–842.
257 Lucas CP, Zabramski JM, Spetzler RF, Jacobowitz R: Treatment for intracranial dural arteriovenous malformations: a meta-analysis from the English language literature. Neurosurgery 1997;40:1119–1132.
258 Ioannidis JPA, Cappelleri JC, Lau J: Issues in comparisons between meta-analyses and large trials. JAMA 1998;279:1089–1093.
259 Bailar JC 3rd: The promise and problems of meta-analysis. N Engl J Med 1997;337:559–561.
260 Naylor CD: Meta-analysis and the meta-epidemiology of clinical research. BMJ 1997;315: 617–619.
261 Eysenck HJ: Meta-analysis or best-evidence synthesis? J Eval Clin Pract 1995;1:29–36.
262 Thompson SG: Why sources of heterogeneity in meta-analysis should be investigated. BMJ 1994;309:1351–1355.
263 Basinski AS, Naylor CD: Further thoughts on the importance of models in the assessment of clinical evidence. J Clin Epidemiol 1992;45:729–732.
264 Egger M, Smith GD: Misleading meta-analysis. BMJ 1995;310:752–754.

265 Villar J, Carroli G, Belizan JM: Predictive ability of meta-analyses of randomized controlled trials. Lancet 1995;345:772–776.
266 Cappelleri JC, Ioannidis JP, Schmid CH, de Ferranti SD, Aubert M, Chalmers TC, Lau J: Large trials vs meta-analysis of smaller trials: how do their results compare? JAMA 1996;276:1332–1338.
267 Charlton BG: Statistical malpractice. J R Coll Physicians Lond 1996;30:112–114.
268 LeLorier J, Gregoire G, Benhaddad A, Lapierre J, Derderian F: Discrepancies between meta-analyses and subsequent large randomized, controlled trials. N Engl J Med 1997;337:536–542.
269 Lau J, Ioannidis JP, Schmid CH: Summing up evidence: one answer is not always enough. Lancet 1998;351:123–127.
270 Teo KK, Yusuf S, Collins R, Held PH, Peto R: Effects of intravenous magnesium in suspected acute myocardial infarction: an overview of randomized trials. BMJ 1991;303:1499–1503.
271 ISIS-4 (Fourth International Study of Infarct Survival Collaborative Group): A randomized factorial trial assessing early oral captopril oral mononitrate, and intravenous magnesium sulphate in 50,050 patients with suspected acute myocardial infarction. Lancet 1995;345:669–685.
272 Linde K, Clausius N, Ramirez G, Melchart D, Eitel F, Hedges LV, Jonas WB: Are the clinical effects of homeopathy placebo effects? A meta-analysis of placebo-controlled trials. Lancet 1997; 350:834–843.
273 Kjaergard LL, Villumsen J, Gluud C: Reported methodologic quality and discrepancies between large and small randomized trials in meta-analyses. Ann Intern Med 2001;135:982–989.
274 Fleiss JL: Statistical Methods for Rates and Proportions, ed 2. New York, Wiley, 1981, pp 260–280.
275 Julian D: Trials and tribulations. Cardiovasc Res 1994;28:598–603.
276 Charlton BG: Megatrials are based on a methodological mistake. Br J Gen Pract 1996;46: 429–431.
277 Charlton DG: The future of clinical research: from megatrials towards methodological rigour and representative sampling. J Eval Clin Pract 1996;2:159–169.
278 Altman DG, Dore CJ: Randomisation and baseline comparisons in clinical trials. Lancet 1990; 335:149–153.
279 Davidson RA: Source of funding and outcome of clinical trials. J Gen Intern Med 1986;1: 155–158.
280 Ioannidis JPA, Lau J: Uncontrolled pearls, controlled evidence, meta-analysis and the individual patient. J Clin Epidemiol 1998;51:709–711.
281 Frankford DM: Scientism and economism in the regulation of health care. J Health Polit Policy Law 1994;19:773–799.
282 Liberati A, Pistotti V, Telaro E: Evidence-based medicine and practice: what's new for the physicians? Forum 1999;9:361–371.
283 Stradling JR, Davies RJ: The unacceptable face of evidence-based medicine. J Eval Clin Pract 1997;3:99–103.
284 Sanders MH, Moore SE, Eveslag J: CPAP via nasal mask: a treatment for occlusive sleep apnea. Chest 1983;83:144–145.
285 Bricolo A, Pasut L: Extradural hematoma: toward zero mortality. A prospective study. Neurosurgery 1984;14:8–12.
286 Cohen J, Montero A, Israel Z: Prognosis and clinical relevance of anisocoria-craniotomy latency for epidural hematoma in comatose patients. J Trauma 1996;41:120–122.
287 Royal College of General Practitioners: The Development and Implementation of Clinical Guidelines: Report of the Clinical Guidelines Working Group. Report from Practice 26. London, Royal College of General Practitioners, 1995.
288 Purves I: Computerised guidelines in primary health care: reflections and implications. Stud Health Technol Inform 1995;16:57–74.
289 Griffiths M: Evidence based medicine. Must be applied critically. BMJ 1995;311:257.
290 Bero LA, Grilli R, Grimshaw JM, Harvey E, Oxman AD, Thomson MA: Closing the gap between research and practice: an overview of systematic reviews of interventions to promote the implementation of research findings. The Cochrane Effective Practice and Organization of Care Review Group. BMJ 1998;317:465–468.
291 National Health Service Centre for Reviews and Dissemination: Getting evidence into practice. Eff Health Care 1999;5:1–15.

292 Style A: Intuition and problem solving. J R Coll Gen Pract 1979;29:71–74.
293 Schmidt HG, Norman GR, Boshuizen HP: A cognitive perspective on medical expertise: theory and implication. Acad Med 1990;65:611–621.
294 Clare A: National variations in medical practice. BMJ 1989;298:1334.
295 Kuhn TS: The Structure of Scientific Revolutions. Chicago, University of Chicago Press, 1970.
296 Wiebe S, Demaerschalk B: Evidence based care in the neurosciences. Can J Neurol Sci 2002;29: 115–119.
297 Grol R: Implementing guidelines in general practice care. Qual Health Care 1992;1:184–191.
298 Haines A, Jones R: Implementing findings of research. BMJ 1994;308:1488–1492.

Mark E. Linskey, MD, Associate Professor and Chairman
Department of Neurological Surgery
Bldg 56, Suite 400, UCI Medical Center
101 The City Drive South
Orange, CA 92868-3298 (USA)
Tel. +1 714 456 6966, Fax +1 714 456 8212, E-Mail mlinskey@uci.edu

Pollock BE (ed): Guiding Neurosurgery by Evidence.
Prog Neurol Surg. Basel, Karger, 2006, vol 19, pp 54–79

Evaluation of Epidemiologic Evidence for Primary Adult Brain Tumor Risk Factors Using Evidence-Based Medicine

James L. Fisher[a,b], *Judith A. Schwartzbaum*[b,c,f], *Margaret Wrensch*[d], *Mitchel S. Berger*[e]

[a]The Arthur G. James Cancer Hospital and Richard J. Solove Research Institute, [b]Comprehensive Cancer Center, [c]Division of Epidemiology and Biometrics, School of Public Health, The Ohio State University, Columbus, Ohio, [d]Departments of Neurological Surgery and Epidemiology and Biostatistics, [e]Department of Neurological Surgery and Brain Tumor Research Center, University of California, San Francisco, Calif., USA; [f]Institute of Environmental Medicine, Karolinska Institute, Stockholm, Sweden

Abstract

We evaluate genetic, behavioral, developmental and experiential risk factors for primary adult brain tumors (primarily, astrocytoma and meningioma) using a systematic set of principles adapted from evidence-based medicine standards. In addition to ionizing radiation, rare mutations in highly penetrant genes associated with certain diseases/syndromes, and epilepsy and seizures (which probably result from, rather than cause, adult brain tumors), only the unexplained observation of familial aggregation of astrocytoma has been consistently shown. There is promising renewed interest in associations between infections, allergic conditions and adult brain tumor risk. Our knowledge of the causes of adult brain tumors is limited and should be expanded by results from large, well-designed studies of novel potential risk factors and potential interactions between known and suspected risk factors.

The purpose of the present review is to evaluate epidemiologic literature concerning risk factors for primary adult brain tumors (ABT) using a standard, systematic set of rules for evaluation. Principles from evidence-based medicine are useful in this regard because they are based on unambiguous guidelines, and because they are understood, accepted and used by many clinicians, researchers,

Table 1. Traditional levels of evidence quality and adaptation for epidemiologic studies of potential primary brain tumor risk factors

Level	Traditional evidence-based medicine classification scheme	Evidence-based medicine classification scheme adapted for epidemiologic studies of potential primary brain tumor risk factors
1	Prospective, randomized, controlled clinical trial with masked outcome assessment, and all of the following: (1) clearly defined outcomes, (2) clearly defined inclusion/exclusion criteria, (3) adequate accounting for (and minimal potential for bias from) dropouts and crossovers, and (4) equivalent baseline characteristics among treatment groups (or statistical adjustment for lack of equivalency)	Prospective cohort study in a representative population, with all of the following: (1) clearly defined outcomes, (2) clearly defined inclusion/exclusion criteria, (3) adequate accounting for (and minimal potential for bias from) dropouts and crossovers, and (4) equivalent baseline characteristics among treatment groups (or statistical adjustment for lack of equivalency)
2	Randomized, controlled clinical trial lacking one of the four characteristics above, or prospective cohort study in a representative population with masked outcome assessment, and meeting the above four criteria	Prospective cohort study in a representative population, lacking one of the four characteristics above, retrospective cohort study in a representative population lacking no more than one of the four characteristics above, or case-control study in a representative population, with adequate control selection, and meeting numbers (1) and (2) above
3	Case-control study	Cohort or case-control study not meeting criteria described for level of evidence quality 2
4	Other study types, including case series, case report, or expert opinion	Other study types, including case series, case report, or expert opinion

policy makers and public health practitioners [1–3]. Because the scheme used to classify levels of evidence in traditional evidence-based medicine was designed, and is predominantly used, for studies intended to examine the efficacy of treatments, as shown in table 1, the highest traditional level of evidence quality (level 1) is assigned to a well-designed prospective, randomized, controlled, clinical trial. However, the primary goal of analytic epidemiology is to understand the causes or risk factors for diseases. Because it is unethical to assign study participants to receive a potentially harmful exposure, clinical trials are not used to evaluate factors that may increase ABT risk. As a result, there is no 'level 1' level of evidence quality, per se, for ABT risk factors (although, in the future, randomized trials of potentially preventive factors such as nonsteroidal anti-inflammatory drugs may be conducted) [4]. Epidemiologic studies usually compare either ABT risk in participants with and without certain characteristics (cohort studies), or the histories of participants with and without ABT (case-control studies). Therefore, a well-designed cohort study, in which groups of participants with and without the potential risk factor are followed over time for the occurrence of ABT, may be considered the highest level of *obtainable* evidence. As shown in table 1, for purposes of the present evaluation, we adapted the levels of evidence quality scheme to consider our epidemiologic goal of understanding the causes of ABT. The primary difference in this adapted scheme is the removal of the randomized, controlled, clinical trial; the level of evidence from the well-designed cohort study is, in our adapted scheme, the superior source of evidence. In addition, it should be noted that because a case-control study utilizing incident cases only differs from a cohort study by the method of sampling controls or noncases, results from a well-designed case-control study often provide nearly as high a level of evidence as a well-designed cohort study. In this review, the relevant distinction between a cohort and case-control study is that results from a cohort study can provide evidence that the potential cause preceded the effect (or ABT), while results from a case-control study cannot address temporality. Studies described in this review are cohort and case-control studies.

We evaluate the epidemiologic evidence for ABT risk factors as follows: (1) identify epidemiologic studies that address the associations of interest by searching Medline for reports of relevant epidemiologic and laboratory studies, (2) for each study, examine the estimated magnitude and precision of the effect (usually a risk or odds ratio), and its validity based on the relative strengths and weakness of the study design, and potential sources of error and bias in the analysis, (3) assign a level of evidence quality to each study (descriptions of levels of evidence are shown in table 1, adapted from Miyasaki et al. [2]), and (4) assign a grade of recommendation to evaluate the potential association between the risk factor and ABT risk (table 2). Grades of recommendation are intended to summarize the overall degree of evidence for the potential association and are based on the following: homogeneity of results from original epidemiologic studies, magnitude of the potential effect, level of evidence for each epidemiologic study, and thoroughness of the epidemiologic literature in addressing the potential

Table 2. Grades of recommendation based on evidence-based medicine classification scheme adapted for epidemiologic studies of potential primary brain tumor risk factors

Grade	Characteristics
A	Homogenous results from level 1 and 2 studies
B	Majority of results are homogenous from level 1 and 2 studies
C	Heterogeneous results from level 1 and 2 studies, with some indication of either increased or decreased risk associated with factor of interest
D	Inconsistent results with no clear indication of increased or decreased risk associated with factor of interest

association [1–3]. It should be noted that we refer to 'level' as related to strength of study design, and to 'grade' as related to the likelihood of a true association between the risk factor and ABT risk. As a result, it is possible for level 1 evidence to support a grade D association. Grade A association would suggest a high likelihood that the potential risk factor actually alters ABT risk.

In addition to original research, we refer to several recent published reviews of the literature that provide thoughtful interpretations and critiques [5–9]. We examine evidence for the following potential ABT risk factors: rare mutations in penetrant genes, familial aggregation, genetic polymorphisms, mutagen sensitivity, infections, allergies and immune-related conditions, head injury and trauma, epilepsy and seizures, estrogen, diet, tobacco smoking, alcohol, ionizing radiation (IR), cellular telephones and electromagnetic fields. We do not discuss the literature on occupational risk factors because it is vast and inconclusive. Wrensch et al. [9] provide a good summary of this literature.

There is a tremendous amount of histologic heterogeneity in ABT. Definitions and classifications of ABT often differ between studies. As a result, it is sometimes difficult to compare studies of participants with overlapping or exclusive histologic classifications. In some earlier studies, analyses were conducted on all ABT combined, while, in most of the more recent studies, investigators separated malignant ABT (such as astrocytoma) from benign ABT (such as meningioma). Further, some studies have concerned more specific histologies, such as glioblastoma multiforme or oligodendroglioma. Studies of more specific histologies may be ideal because they help to discern the histology-specific nature of potentially causal factors. However, for most risk factors described in this review, the evidence available is limited to glioma (or the subtype, astrocytoma, that includes glioblastoma multiforme, anaplastic astrocytoma and astrocytoma) and meningioma. Therefore, in this review, we present results pertaining to astrocytoma (or subtypes) meningioma, and additional histologic groups, when they are available.

ABT are thought to develop through the progressive accumulation of genetic alterations that permit cells to evade normal regulatory mechanisms and escape destruction by the immune system. The epidemiologic information available concerning genetic factors and ABT risk results from studies relating to the following: (1) ABT risk associated with rare mutations in penetrant genes, (2) patterns of ABT in families (suggesting potential inheritance), and (3) genetic polymorphism or variability. These are discussed separately.

Rare Mutations in Penetrant Genes

Several diseases/syndromes associated with rare mutations in highly penetrant genes increase ABT risk. However, in a population-based study of 500 adults with glioma in San Francisco, Calif. [10], less than 1% had a known hereditary syndrome. While it is thought that genetic predisposition is influential in relatively few brain tumors (5–10%) [11], the proportion may be underestimated because some hereditary syndromes are not readily diagnosed and because patients with ABT are not routinely referred to a clinical geneticist.

In general, there is strong evidence that some genetic diseases or syndromes increase risk of ABT [9, 12]. Among these, the following have been associated with an increased ABT risk: tuberous sclerosis complex, neurofibromatosis types 1 and 2 [13], nevoid basal cell carcinoma syndrome, syndromes related to adenomatous polyps and Li-Fraumeni cancer family syndrome [9, 12]. Inherited p53 germline mutations, characteristic of Li-Fraumeni syndrome, are important in the development of many cancers, including ABT [14–16]. In addition, germline p53 mutations have been more frequently found in patients who have multifocal glioma, glioma and another primary malignancy, or a family history of cancer than in patients with other brain tumors [17].

Overall grade of recommendation: A, for association between genetic diseases/syndromes related to rare mutations in highly penetrant genes and ABT risk.

Familial Aggregation

Although a few epidemiologic studies have addressed the potential familial aggregation of meningioma [18–20], results are limited, compared to those concerning glioma and its most common subtype, astrocytic tumors. Among meningioma patients, the standardized incidence ratio (SIR) for having a parent with any nervous system cancer was 2.5 [19], and 3.1 for having a parent with meningioma [18]. Findings from epidemiologic studies of familial aggregation and glioma risk are relatively consistent, although the estimates of the magnitude of increased risk as a result of first degree relation are widely variable [10, 18, 19, 21–29]. Five case-control studies suggest the presence of familial aggregation of glioma or glioma subtypes [10, 21, 22, 28, 29], while one case-control study suggests otherwise [27]. The finding of an increased astrocytoma or glioma risk as a result of familial aggregation is also supported by the analyses of six Swedish cohorts, although these studies contain overlapping populations [18, 19, 23, 25, 26, 30]. Malmer et al. [26] suggest that approximately 2% of glioma cases may be explained by an autosomal recessive gene, although a polygenic model could not be rejected, and that approximately 5% of glioma cases are familial. In a population-based case-control study, Malmer et al. [24] report that, among 37 familial glioma cases (compared to 58 sporadic glioma controls with no family history of glioma), familial cases had more p53-negative tumors. Segregation analyses of families of more than 600 adult patients with glioma showed that a polygenic model best explained the pattern of occurrence of brain tumors [31].

Because it is possible that common environmental exposures experienced by families, in addition to their genetic characteristics, may result in a greater familial ABT risk, several studies have tried to determine whether genetic or environmental factors explain the increased familial risk. Grossman et al. [32] showed that ABT occur in families with no known predisposing hereditary disease and that the pattern of occurrence in many families suggests environmental causes. However, results from a cohort study conducted by Malmer et al. [25] suggest that first-degree relatives, and not spouses, have a significantly increased ABT risk. Therefore, it is likely that genetic characteristics play a role in familial aggregation of ABT.

Although the strength of evidence for familial aggregation of glioma or its subtypes varies among studies, evidence for the presence of familial aggregation has been consistently observed in both cohort and case-control studies. Evidence pertaining to familial aggregation of meningioma is limited and should be validated through additional studies; however, there is weak evidence for the presence of familial aggregation of meningioma.

Overall grade of recommendation: A, for presence of familial aggregation of astrocytoma evaluated separately or for glioma as a whole.

Overall grade of recommendation: C, for presence of familial aggregation of meningioma.

Genetic Polymorphisms

Available evidence suggests that only a small proportion of primary brain tumors result from effects of inherited rare mutations in highly penetrant genes;

therefore, investigators have turned their attention to polymorphisms in genes that might influence susceptibility to brain tumors in concert with environmental exposures. Genetic alterations that affect oxidative metabolism, detoxification of carcinogens, DNA stability and repair, or immune response are candidates, which might plausibly confer genetic susceptibility to ABT.

Results from case-control studies of genes that detoxify carcinogens are inconsistent. For example, case-control studies suggest both that cytochrome P450 2D6 (CYP2D6) increases both astrocytoma (OR = 4.17, p = 0.0043) and meningioma (OR = 4.90, p = 0.0132) risks [33], and that individuals with a poor metabolizer CYP2D6 variant allele are at no greater ABT risk [34]. In two additional case-control studies, Trizna et al. [35] found no association between the null genotype of CYP1A1 and risk of glioma in adults, but De Roos et al. [36] found that CYP2E1 *Rsa*I variant was associated with glioma (OR = 1.4, 95% CI: 0.9–2.4) and acoustic neuroma (OR = 2.3, 95% CI: 1.0–5.3) risks, especially among younger cases.

Detoxifying glutathione S-transferase genes have also been extensively studied and also produce mixed results. Glutathione transferase theta (GSTT1) null genotype appears to increase astrocytoma (OR = 2.67, p = 0.0005) and meningioma (OR = 4.52, p = 0.0001) risks [33]. Results reported by Hand et al. [37] support these findings for astrocytoma, especially high grade astrocytoma, but results reported by Kelsey et al. [34] suggest no association between the GSTT1 null genotype and astrocytoma risk. However, the oligodendroglioma risk was associated with the GSTT1 null genotype (OR = 3.2, 95% CI: 1.1–9.2). Trizna et al. [35] and De Roos et al. [36] report no associations between the null genotype of GSTT1 and glioma risk; however, results reported by De Roos et al. suggest that GSTT1 null genotype increases meningioma risk (OR = 1.5, 95% CI: 1.0–2.3), and that the GSTP1 105 Val/Val genotype is associated with increased glioma risk (OR = 1.8, 95% CI: 1.2–2.7), with evidence of a dose-response trend with an increasing number of variant alleles. Most recently, Wrensch et al. [38] found little evidence for the association of glutathione S-transferase polymorphism with glioma histologic variants.

Several additional polymorphisms have been evaluated for their relationship with glioma. Chen et al. [39] showed that AA or AC versus CC genotype in nucleotide 8092 of ERCC1 increased the oligoastrocytoma risk (OR = 4.6, 95% CI: 1.6–13.2). Caggana et al. [40] found the AA genotype (C to A polymorphism [R156R]) of ERCC2 was more prevalent than the CC or CA genotypes in cases with glioblastoma multiforme, astrocytoma, or oligoastrocytoma than in controls, and the association was strongest for oligoastrocytoma (OR = 3.2, 95% CI: 1.1–9.5). Inconsistencies among genetic polymorphism studies may result from false-positive associations based on inadequate sample sizes [41] and from confounding by genes with similar functions not accounted for in the analyses. Another possibility may be that study populations consist of different proportions of types of tumors, and genetic risk for certain subtypes could be masked by a lack of risk among other subtypes. When these issues are addressed, the potential interaction between genetic polymorphisms with other genetic characteristics and environmental factors can be properly evaluated.

Overall grade of recommendation: C, for association between genetic polymorphisms and ABT risk.

Mutagen Sensitivity

Bondy et al. [42] found that lymphocyte mutagen sensitivity to gamma radiation appears to increase glioma risk. Lymphocytes from glioma patients, compared to those from matched controls, are more sensitive to gamma radiation [42]. Bondy et al. [42] observed a greater frequency of chromatid breaks per cell among glioma patients, compared to controls, and mutagen sensitivity was found to be associated with increased glioma risk (OR = 2.09, 95% CI: 1.43–3.06). Further, there was evidence of a statistically significant dose-response trend between frequency of chromatid breaks and glioma risk [42]. However, because Bondy et al. used the case-control design, it is not possible to determine whether chromatid breaks increased ABT risk or represent a systemic effect of the tumors themselves [43]. To definitively establish temporality, further studies of mutagen sensitivity need to be conducted on blood from glioma patients collected before glioma initiation and development.

Overall grade of recommendation: B, for association between mutagen sensitivity and glioma risk.

Infections

Infection with viruses, such as simian virus 40 (SV40) and varicella zoster virus (VZV), and nonviral infectious agents, such as *Toxoplasma gondii*, or immunity to these agents might influence ABT risk, although the potential risk from these agents has been inadequately addressed in epidemiologic studies. Between 1955 and 1963, an unknown proportion of all inactivated and live polio vaccines distributed was contaminated with SV40 [44]. In Germany, children were followed over a 20-year period, and those inoculated with the polio vaccine contaminated with SV40 had higher occurrences of glioblastoma multiforme, medulloblastoma, and some less common brain tumor types than those not given the contaminated vaccine [45]; in the US, on the other hand, no difference in ABT risk was found for major ABT types (glioma and meningioma) between the two groups of children [46], but one study reported that the incidence of ependymoma was 37% greater among the children receiving the contaminated vaccine [44]. Results from one case-control study suggest that prior infection with VZV, either based on self-report [47] or serologic evidence [48], may be inversely associated with adult glioma risk. In addition, there is mixed evidence from laboratory studies concerning the involvement of JC virus [49–54], BK virus [49, 50, 52], SV40 [49, 50, 52] and human herpes virus 6 (HHV-6) [55] in the development of ABT. Results from a nested case-control study conducted by Rollison et al. [56] indicated that infection with either JC or BK virus, or SV40, as measured in sera of patients between 1 and 22 years prior to ABT diagnosis, did not significantly increase subsequent ABT risk. The potential role of these viruses in the development of ABT is not fully understood, and should be more thoroughly examined. The potential association between infection with HIV and ABT risk has not been addressed in epidemiologic studies, although it is possible that the incidence of ABT among those infected with HIV is greater than that of the general population [57].

A history of cold or influenza infection appears to decrease glioma risk [58, 59]. In a case-control study, Schlehofer et al. [59] found a 30% reduction in glioma risk from a self-report of a history of colds or influenza infections (RR = 0.72, 95% CI: 0.61–0.85). In another case-control study, Fisher et al. found that treatment for at least one cold or influenza infection between 2 and 5 years prior to diagnosis decreases glioma risk approximately 3-fold (OR = 0.39, 95% CI: 0.18–0.86) [58]. These results should be validated in cohort studies with serologic or symptom-based confirmation of infection.

Antibodies to *T. gondii* have been associated with meningioma in a case-control study [60], and to astrocytoma in another study [61], but not to glioma, based on the results of Ryan et al. [60].

The findings concerning infections and ABT risk are limited, inconsistent or based exclusively on results from case-control studies. The strongest epidemiologic evidence of potential association between infection and ABT risk would be submitted from a cohort study in which serologic measurement of viral or bacterial exposure was ascertained prior to ABT development.

Overall grade of recommendation: C, for association between viral and bacterial infections and ABT risk.

Allergies and Immune-Related Conditions

Several recent reports have suggested that a history of allergies and immune-related conditions, such as asthma, eczema and rheumatoid arthritis, decrease the risk of glioma. Although the mechanism governing such potential protection has not been identified, there is speculation that it may arise from the anti-inflammatory effects of cytokines involved in allergic and autoimmune disease [62–65]. Five case-control studies have reported decreases in glioblastoma multiforme, glioma or astrocytoma risk from allergies and immune-related conditions [22, 59, 62, 65, 66], while results from one case-control study suggest no difference in glioma risk [21]. For example, Brenner et al. [62] reported an inverse association between glioma risk and history of any allergy (OR = 0.67, 95% CI: 0.52–0.86) or autoimmune disease (OR = 0.49, 95% CI: 0.35–0.69). No such decrease in risk for meningioma [59, 62, 66] was observed. A problem with case-control association between reported allergy status and glioma is that due to the low survival probability from glioblastoma mutiforme many proxy respondents were used to ascertain information on allergic conditions. Confirming the suggestion that proxy reports may not be reliable, Schwartzbaum et al. [63] found a correlation between whether a proxy respondent was used and the presence or absence of allergic conditions. Specifically, proxy respondents reported fewer allergic conditions than did self-reporting respondents. However, in a cohort study where information on allergic conditions was obtained on the average at least 19 years before brain tumor diagnosis, Schwartzbaum et al. [63] report results from the first series of cohort studies, consistent with an inverse association between allergies and glioma risk (hazard ratio [HR] = 0.45, 95% CI: 0.19–1.07), although not among low grade glioma, and between immune-related hospital discharges and glioma risk (HR = 0.46, 95% CI: 0.14–1.49). Further suggesting that the association between allergic conditions and glioma risk is not a reporting artifact, Schwartzbaum et al. found that genetic polymorphisms associated with an increased risk of allergic conditions appear to decrease glioma risk (unpubl. observation). Although the majority of results indicate an inverse association between allergies and immune-related conditions and glioma risk, further studies are needed to provide solid evidence.

Overall grade of recommendation: B, for inverse association between allergies, immune-related conditions and glioma, but not meningioma, risk.

Head Injury or Trauma

Head injury and trauma have been examined as potential ABT risk factors in several epidemiologic studies. Compared to glioma, there is slightly stronger evidence that head injury and trauma may increase meningioma risk. Results from four case-control studies suggest that head injury and trauma increase meningioma risk [67–70]. Among males, Preston-Martin et al. [69] found that meningioma was more common among those who reported having ever had a head injury (OR = 1.5, 95% CI: 0.9–2.6), and that, among those with a latency of 15–24 years, meningioma risk was much greater (OR = 5.4, 95% CI: 1.7–16.6). However, these results are in conflict with the results of three cohort studies, which suggest no increase in meningioma risk from head injury or trauma [71–73]. Results from the three cohort studies provide much stronger evidence because it is likely that there were differences between cases and controls in the reporting of previous head injury and trauma [9, 72]. Hu et al. [74] found an increase in glioma risk from head trauma requiring medical attention (OR = 4.1, 95% CI: 2.5–10.3), and Hochberg et al. [75] found a large increase in glioblastoma multiforme risk from severe head injury. However, results from four additional case-control studies, and two cohort studies suggested no such association [9, 29, 68, 69, 72, 73, 76]. A large Danish cohort study provides good evidence that there is little, if any, association between head injury and trauma and either meningioma or glioma risk. Inskip et al. [72] and Wrensch et al. [9] found that, after excluding injuries occurring within the year prior to diagnosis (which could have resulted in tumor detection) neither glioma risk (SIR = 1.0, 95% CI: 0.8–1.2) nor meningioma risk (SIR = 1.2, 95% CI: 0.8–1.7) was elevated. Risk of some intravascular tumors was elevated. However, given that intravascular tumors are far less common than meningioma or glioma, the increase in overall ABT risk from head injury and trauma is probably slight, if existent.

Overall grade of recommendation: D, for association between head injury or trauma and both meningioma and glioma risk.

Overall grade of recommendation: B, for association between head injury or trauma and intravascular tumor risk.

Epilepsy and Seizures

Seizures prior to ABT diagnoses are common [77]. There is relatively consistent evidence from case-control studies that epilepsy or seizure disorders are associated with increased meningioma risk, although not all findings have been statistically significant [59, 66, 78, 79]. The evidence concerning epilepsy or seizure disorders and glioma risk is somewhat stronger. Results from four case-control studies [10, 59, 66, 79] and three cohort studies [78, 80, 81] indicate an increase in glioma risk from a history of epilepsy or seizure. Lamminpaa et al. [78] found an excess of both meningioma and glioma associated with a history of prescription for antiepileptic medication. Schlehofer et al. [59] found an increased glioma risk associated with a history of epilepsy (RR = 6.55, 95% CI: 3.40–12.63), but the relative risk diminished when including only those with epilepsy lasting at least 20 years. Importantly, for glioma, but not meningioma, risk has been shown to increase with proximity to diagnosis and decrease with duration of epilepsy, suggesting that epilepsy is not a cause but rather a result, an early effect, of ABT [79].

Overall grade of recommendation: A, for association between epilepsy and seizures and both meningioma and glioma risk, although epilepsy and seizures probably result from rather than cause ABT.

Estrogen, Reproductive and Menstrual Factors

Epidemiologic evidence indicates that the sex hormone, estrogen, may be associated with increased meningioma risk. Meningioma is approximately twice as common in females [82, 83]. In addition, some meningioma express progesterone receptors [84–86], and this expression occurs to a greater degree among females [86]. Studies of meningioma risk and menopausal status, age at menarche, and parity have produced some results supporting the notion that greater exposure to endogenous estrogen increases meningioma risk and some that have supported the notion that lesser exposure increases meningioma risk. Results from a cohort study suggest that postmenopausal women who have never used estrogen replacement therapy are at greater meningioma risk compared to premenopausal women (RR = 2.48, 95% CI: 1.29–4.77), and the risk remains significantly greater comparing postmenopausal women who have used estrogen replacement therapy to premenopausal women (RR = 1.86, 95% CI: 1.07–3.24) [87]. These results are supported by those of Schlehofer et al. [88] who found that postmenopausal women had a reduced risk of meningioma (RR = 0.58, 95% CI: 0.18–1.90) compared to premenopausal women. Concerning age at menarche, Jhawar et al. [87] found that later age at menarche (after age 14 years) increased meningioma risk (OR = 1.97, 95% CI: 1.06–3.66). Further, there was an increased risk of meningioma among parous women compared to nulliparous women (RR = 2.39, 95% CI: 0.76–7.53). However, findings from two case-control studies suggest no association between parity and meningioma risk [88, 89]. On the whole, there is consistency among results concerning increased meningioma risk among premenopausal women, that is, at a given age, women who are still premenopausal are at higher risk than women who are postmenopausal, suggesting that increased exposure to menstrual hormones might increase risk. However, results concerning parity and age at menarche suggest that estrogen or other reproductive or menstrual hormones might decrease meningioma risk. One would expect parous women and women who started menarche at older ages to have lower meningioma risk, if estrogen increases risk, because parous women and women who started menarche at older ages are exposed to endogenous estrogen for a shorter amount of time. Further study is required to understand hormone-related factors, especially because the findings presented here are statistically significant and opposite to those expected under the hypothesis that estrogen influences meningioma risk. It is also possible that menstrual and reproductive factors alone are not sufficient to accurately classify lifetime estrogen or other hormonal exposure.

Estrogen may also be associated with decreased astrocytoma risk. Astrocytoma is approximately 40% more common among males [9]. A study of the incidence of astrocytoma subtypes occurring in the State of New York suggests that, for glioblastoma multiforme, the protective effect of female sex occurs between the approximate ages of menarche and menopause, and that this protection decreases in postmenopausal age groups [90]. Schlehofer et al. [88] report that postmenopausal women whose menopause was not surgically induced are at greater risk of glioma and acoustic neuroma, although the finding was not statistically significant. However, like the association with meningioma, the association between estrogen and astrocytoma risk may not be straightforward. For example, results from two case-control studies suggest that astrocytoma risk [91] and risk of the subtypes glioma [89] and glioblastoma multiforme [91] are lower among parous women. Schlehofer et al. [88] report no association between parity and glioma risk.

For both meningioma and astrocytoma, estrogen, and perhaps other hormones, may alter risks. However, the results do not support the notion that the longer the duration of exogenous estrogen exposure the greater the risk. Cohort studies of ABT risk among women who have and have not taken estrogen replacement therapy should be conducted.

Overall grade of recommendation: B, for associations between reproductive and menstrual factors and estrogen and both meningioma and astrocytoma risk, although the associations are not straightforward.

Diet

Three groups of diet-related risk factors have emerged as potentially affecting ABT risk. These are N-nitroso compounds, antioxidant intake and calcium intake. They are discussed separately.

N-Nitroso Compounds

N-nitroso compounds (especially nitrosamides) are potent neurocarcinogens. Assessing exposure to N-nitroso compounds is difficult because they are common in both endogenous and exogenous sources, including food. Vegetables that are high in nitrites also contain vitamins that may block the formation of N-nitroso compounds. Cured meats contain nitrites, which are precursors of

N-nitroso compounds. Results from epidemiologic studies concerning ABT risk associated with cured meat consumption are mixed. Results from a case-control study of cured meat consumption and meningioma risk suggest an increase ABT risk, but only for females [92], while two case-controls studies report conflicting evidence of the effect of cured meat consumption on glioma risk, one reporting no effect [93], and one reporting that male cases, but not female cases, were more likely than controls to report higher levels of cured meat consumption [94]. However, as suggested by Schwartzbaum et al. [95], it is possible that energy intake and γ-tocopherol modify the association between cured meat consumption and glioma risk. (Cured meats have a high-energy and low-γ-tocopherol content.) A recent meta-analysis [96] was conducted of nine studies addressing the possible association between cured meat consumption and glioma risk, and although an increase in glioma risk was found from cured meat consumption (pooled RR = 1.48, 95% CI: 1.20–1.83), Huncharek et al. point out that individual studies failed to adjust for potential confounding by energy intake. In a small-area ecologic study of England, a higher incidence of ABT was found in areas with greater nitrate content in drinking water [97].

Antioxidant Intake

Oxidative stress results from excessive accumulation of reactive oxygen species, and can be caused by inadequate dietary antioxidant intake. Antioxidants are abundant in a diet high in fruits and vegetables. Consumption of greater amounts of vitamin C was inversely associated with glioma risk in two case-control studies [94, 98], although the findings were statistically significant only among males in the study conducted by Lee et al. [94]. Schwartzbaum et al. [95] found lower levels of vitamin C intake among glioma cases compared to controls. The results reported by Chen et al. [39], however, suggest no association between vitamin C intake and glioma risk. Dietary intake of higher levels of vitamin A or provitamin A has been inversely related to glioma risk in each of three case-control studies in which it was examined [93, 94, 98], although not all findings were statistically significant. Higher levels of dietary vitamin E intake were found to be protective for glioma in one case-control study [98], but not in two other studies [93, 94]. Schwartzbaum et al. [95] found lower levels of vitamin E (both α- and γ-tocopherol) intake among glioma cases compared to controls.

Calcium Intake

Dietary calcium may decrease glioma risk through increasing apoptosis, promoting DNA repair, and decreasing the production of parathyroid hormone [99]. Tedeschi-Blok et al. [99] found greater levels of calcium intake to protect against glioma, but only among females. The results of another case-control study suggest that calcium is protective for all ABT combined [98].

Evidence related to dietary factors is inconsistent and remains limited. Further study is needed to examine these factors and their potential interaction with one another, as well as other potential ABT risk factors.

Overall grade of recommendation: C, for association between consumption of N-nitroso compounds, and antioxidant and calcium intakes and ABT risk.

Tobacco Smoking

Tobacco smoking has been evaluated as a potential risk factor for ABT because some carcinogenic components contained in tobacco smoke, including nitroso compounds, penetrate the blood-brain barrier. A case-control study showed no increase in glioblastoma multiforme risk from tobacco smoking [22]. However, results from two case-control studies suggest that there may be a difference between males and females in the association between tobacco smoking and glioma risk. In one study, males, but not females, who reported a history of having ever smoked were at greater risk of glioma [100], while results from another study suggest that among men only, cases were almost 2 times more likely to report smoking unfiltered cigarettes [94]. Tobacco smoking has been shown to increase meningioma risk, but only in females [101]. Results from most studies suggest that tobacco smoking does not strongly contribute to ABT risk, although smoking unfiltered, but not filtered, cigarettes may increase glioma risk [94]. Overall, the results are inconsistent and the magnitudes of the effect estimates are modest.

Overall grade of recommendation: D, for association between filtered cigarette smoking and glioma and meningioma risk. C, for association between unfiltered cigarette smoking and glioma risk.

Alcohol

Results from seven case-control studies addressing alcohol consumption and ABT risk are inconsistent, with five studies suggesting no increase in ABT risk [22, 66, 100, 101, 102], and two suggesting modest increases in risk [74, 94]. Alcohol consumption has not been shown to affect meningioma risk [66, 101, 102], and glioma risk was found to be increased from higher levels of alcohol consumption in one study [74, 94], while, in four other studies, there was no increase in glioma risk [66, 100, 102], or glioblastoma multiforme risk [22]. Overall, the results are inconsistent and the magnitudes of the positive results are modest.

Overall grade of recommendation: D, for association between alcohol consumption and glioma and meningioma risk.

Ionizing Radiation

Therapeutic IR may be the strongest modifiable ABT risk factor [8, 9]. IR used to treat tinea capitis and skin hemangioma in children or infants has been associated with relative risks of 18 for nerve sheath tumors, 10 for meningioma, and 3 for glioma [8, 9]. Twelve reports of original studies concerning exposure to IR were reviewed. Results from two studies concerning exposure to cosmic IR from occupation as a pilot or aircrew/cockpit crew member revealed no elevation in ABT risk [103, 104]. Results from two cohort studies indicated that occupation involving working with nuclear materials increases ABT risk, apparently as a result of IR exposure [105, 106]. However, it is difficult to rule out the possibility that these results are confounded by chemical exposures occurring in nuclear industry occupations. Exposure to nondental X-rays of the head and neck did not increase glioma risk in one case-control study [76], but both radiotherapy of the head and neck and diagnostic X-rays were found to increase ABT risk in another case-control study [107]. Prior radiotherapy is relatively common (17%) among patients with glioblastoma multiforme [108], and results from several studies have suggested increases in risk of glioma and other ABT from a history of radiotherapy for acute lymphoblastic leukemia as children [109, 110]. Second primary brain tumors also occur more frequently than expected, especially among patients treated with radiotherapy [111].

Studies of ABT risk and dental X-rays are less abundant. Results from one case-control study suggest that only exposure to full-mouth (and not bitewing, lateral cephalometric, or panoramic) X-rays performed 15–40 years prior to diagnosis increases meningioma risk [112]. These results are supported by another study suggesting that the meningioma risk is more strongly associated with exposures from dental X-rays taken in the more distant past.

A study of survivors of the atomic bombing of Hiroshima showed a high incidence of meningioma correlating with the dose of radiation to the brain [113]. The incidence increased with closer proximity to the hypocenter. Japanese studies of atomic bomb survivors have not shown an increased risk of ABT among those who were exposed in utero [8].

On the whole, results from studies of the association between IR exposure and ABT risk are homogenous.

Overall grade of recommendation: A, for association between IR and glioma and meningioma risk.

Cellular Telephones

Because of public concern over possible health effects associated with cellular telephone use, several studies have addressed the potential association between use of cellular telephones and ABT risk. Of these, one mortality study [114], four case-control studies [115–118] and one retrospective cohort study [119] suggest that there is no association between cellular telephone use and ABT risk. Further, results from these studies, in general, suggest that there is no increase in ABT risk from longer duration of cellular telephone use and that there is no specific anatomic site or ABT histology affected by these devices. However, three reports provide additional important findings. Results reported by Hardell et al. [107] suggest an increase in ABT risk from ipsilateral (same side) use of cellular telephones for areas of the brain with the greatest potential for microwave exposure from cellular telephone use (temporal, temporoparietal and occipital areas). Moreover, ipsilateral radiofrequency exposure was associated with an increase in *malignant* ABT risk, although the association was stronger for analog, versus digital, radiofrequency; for astrocytoma, risk was nearly double [120]. (Analog cellular telephone radiofrequency signals operate in the range of 800–900 MHz, while newer digital phones operate in the range of 1,600–2,000 MHz.) Further, similar results concerning ipsilateral cellular telephone use were reported in a recent case-control study, and statistically significant increases in ABT risk, including astrocytoma risk, were found for both analog and digital devices, although, again, the finding was stronger for analog devices [121]. There has been no known association reported for use of cellular telephones on the opposite side of the brain.

Although results are inconsistent, if there is an increase in ABT risk from cellular telephone use, it may be specific to ipsilateral use, especially from analog telephones, and especially for anatomic areas of the brain near the device. Although results from most known studies of cellular telephones and ABT, on the whole, suggest no increase in ABT risk, it is important to continue this line of study because: (1) the use of such devices is increasingly common, and (2) it is possible that adverse health effects from this exposure may result from *long-term* exposure, and due to the recent increase in cellular telephone usage, it is possible that results from many studies have not accounted for the possible long lag time between exposure and ABT, especially slow-growing ABT. In addition, changes in cellular telephone technology, such as the predominance of digital, versus analog, telephones, as well as an overall increase in the duration of usage, could not be addressed in many studies.

Overall grade of recommendation: C, for association between cellular telephone use and ABT risk.

Electromagnetic Fields

Concern over exposure to low-frequency electric and magnetic fields (EMF) has stimulated considerable public and scientific attention. Primarily, this interest arises from residential studies showing increased risks of brain tumors and leukemia in children whose homes have high EMF exposures. However, for ABT, exposure to EMF has, for the most part, been evaluated through occupational studies of workers presumably exposed to greater levels of EMF. In general, workers exposed to greater levels of EMF have higher incidence and mortality rates of ABT. Twenty-one reports of original occupational studies were reviewed. In general, results from each of the 11 case-control studies addressing occupational EMF exposure and ABT risk suggest an increase in ABT risk associated with greater levels of EMF exposure, although not every increase in risk was statistically significant [122–132]. Results from nested case-control and cohort studies have yielded inconsistent results, with five suggesting no association [133–137], and five suggesting an increase in ABT risk from occupational exposure to EMF [124, 138–141]. In studies of specific histologic types, risk for the following types of ABT was increased with occupational exposure to EMF: astrocytoma [124, 126], glioma [122, 132], or glioblastoma multiforme [131, 140]. The relationship between occupational EMF exposure and ABT risk may not be straightforward. For example, results from a recent study suggest that occupational exposure to high levels of EMF may be associated with glioma, but not meningioma, risk in the presence of carcinogenic chemicals [140]. That is, EMF may modify the association between occupational chemical exposures and glioma, but not meningioma, risk. Residential exposure to EMF has been examined by Wrensch et al. [142], and results from this study did not support an association between residential exposure to EMF and ABT risk. No causal relationship has been established between exposure to EMF, either occupational or residential, and ABT risk.

Studies of exposure to EMF and ABT risk may be flawed by the difficulty of assessing the potentially imperceptible and ubiquitous exposure, and by not knowing the period during which exposure assessment should be determined, given the absence of available information about the time period between exposure and ABT risk. It is likely that studies of EMF exposure and ABT risk have been flawed by large exposure misclassification. There is no established and accepted mechanism of action by which exposure to EMF may increase ABT risk. There is inconsistency of results across studies, and an apparent lack of dose-response (although it is possible that a threshold value exists above which ABT risk is affected).

Overall grade of recommendation: C, for association between EMF exposure and ABT risk.

Table 3. Potential primary brain tumor risk factors and corresponding grades of recommendation based on an evidence-based medicine classification scheme adapted for epidemiologic studies

Potential primary brain tumor risk factor	Grade of recommendation
Genetic characteristics	
Diseases/syndromes associated with rare mutations	A
Familial aggregation for astrocytoma (and subtypes)	A
Familial aggregation for meningioma	C
Genetic polymorphisms	C
Mutagen sensitivity	B
Nongenetic characteristics	
Infections	C
Allergies and immune-related conditions for glioma	B
Head injury and trauma	D
Head injury and trauma for intravascular tumors	B
Epilepsy and seizures (although probably not causes)	A
Estrogen, reproductive and menstrual factors	B
Diet (N-nitroso compounds, antioxidants, calcium)	C
Tobacco smoking	
Unfiltered cigarettes	C
Filtered cigarettes	D
Alcohol consumption	D
IR	A
Cellular telephone use	C
EMF	C

Conclusion

As can be seen in table 3, there are few established risk factors for ABT. In addition to IR, rare mutations in highly penetrant genes associated with certain diseases/syndromes, and epilepsy and seizures (which probably result from, rather than cause, ABT), only the unexplained observation of familial aggregation has been consistently shown. Rather than examining individual genetic polymorphisms, present research is focused on genetic polymorphisms in metabolic pathways involved in carcinogenesis. Related pathways are also studied simultaneously so that confounding by genes with similar functions can be avoided. Large sample sizes are required for such studies and these larger studies avoid false-positive findings and allow examination of the modifying effects of polymorphisms on environmental exposures, as well as the potential for interaction between germline mutations and sporadic tumor mutations. In addition, there is renewed interest in the association between infections, allergic conditions and ABT risk. Our knowledge of the causes of ABT is limited and should be expanded by results from large, well-designed studies of novel potential risk factors and potential interactions between known and suspected risk factors.

References

1 Jenicek M: Epidemiology, evidenced-based medicine, and evidence-based public health. J Epidemiol 1997;7:187–197.
2 Miyasaki JM, Martin W, Suchowersky O, Weiner WJ, Lang AE: Practice parameter: initiation of treatment for Parkinson's disease: an evidence-based review: report of the Quality Standards Subcommittee of the American Academy of Neurology. Neurology 2002;58:11–17.
3 Spector R, Vesell ES: The pursuit of clinical truth: role of epidemiology/observation studies. J Clin Pharmacol 2000;40:1205–1210.
4 Sivak-Sears N, Schwartzbaum J, Miike R, Moghadassi M, Wrensch M: Case-control study of non-steroidal anti-inflammatory drug use and glioblastoma multiforme. Am J Epidemiol, in press.
5 Aldape KD, Okcu MF, Bondy ML, Wrensch M: Molecular epidemiology of glioblastoma. Cancer J 2003;9:99–106.
6 Gurney JG, Kadan-Lottick N: Brain and other central nervous system tumors: rates, trends, and epidemiology. Curr Opin Oncol 2001;13:160–166.
7 Inskip PD, Linet MS, Heineman EF: Etiology of brain tumors in adults. Epidemiol Rev 1995;17: 382–414.
8 Preston-Martin S: Epidemiology of primary CNS neoplasms. Neurol Clin 1996;14:273–290.
9 Wrensch M, Minn Y, Chew T, Bondy M, Berger MS: Epidemiology of primary brain tumors: current concepts and review of the literature. Neurooncology 2002;4:278–299.
10 Wrensch M, Lee M, Miike R, Newman B, Barger G, Davis R, Wiencke J, Neuhaus J: Familial and personal medical history of cancer and nervous system conditions among adults with glioma and controls. Am J Epidemiol 1997;145:581–593.
11 Narod SA, Stiller C, Lenoir GM: An estimate of the heritable fraction of childhood cancer. Br J Cancer 1991;63:993–999.
12 Bondy M, Wiencke J, Wrensch M, Kyritsis AP: Genetics of primary brain tumors: a review. J Neurooncol 1994;18:69–81.
13 Huson SM, Harper PS, Compston DA: Von Recklinghausen neurofibromatosis. A clinical and population study in south-east Wales. Brain 1988;111:1355–1381.
14 Akashi M, Koeffler HP: Li-Fraumeni syndrome and the role of the p53 tumor suppressor gene in cancer susceptibility. Clin Obstet Gynecol 1998;41:172–199.
15 Malkin D: p53 and the Li-Fraumeni syndrome. Cancer Genet Cytogenet 1993;66:83–92.
16 Nichols KE, Malkin D, Garber JE, Fraumeni JFJ, Li FP: Germ-line p53 mutations predispose to a wide spectrum of early-onset cancers. Cancer Epidemiol Biomarkers Prev 2001;10:83–87.
17 Kyritsis AP, Bondy ML, Xiao M, Berman EL, Cunningham JE, Lee PS, Levin VA, Saya H: Germline p53 gene mutations in subsets of glioma patients. J Natl Cancer Inst 1994;86:344–349.
18 Hemminki K, Li X: Familial risks in nervous system tumors. Cancer Epidemiol Biomarkers Prev 2003;12:1137–1142.
19 Hemminki K, Li X, Collins VP: Parental cancer as a risk factor for brain tumors (Sweden). Cancer Causes Control 2001;12:195–199.
20 Paunu N, Pukkala E, Laippala P, Sankila R, Isola J, Miettinen H, Simola KOJ, Helen P, Helin H, Haapasalo H: Cancer incidence in families with multiple glioma patients. Int J Cancer 2002;97: 819–822.
21 Cicuttini FM, Hurley SF, Forbes A, Donnan GA, Salzberg M, Giles GG, McNeil JJ: Association of adult glioma with medical conditions, family and reproductive history. Int J Cancer 1997;71: 203–207.

22 Hochberg F, Toniolo P, Cole P, Salcman M: Nonoccupational risk indicators of glioblastoma in adults. J Neurooncol 1990;8:55–60.
23 Malmer B, Gronberg H, Bergenheim AT, Lenner P, Henriksson R: Familial aggregation of astrocytoma in northern Sweden: an epidemiological cohort study. Int J Cancer 1999;81:366–370.
24 Malmer B, Brannstrom T, Andersson U, Bergh K, Gronberg H, Henriksson R: Does a low frequency of P53 and Pgp expression in familial glioma compared to sporadic controls indicate biological differences? Anticancer Res 2002;22:3949–3954.
25 Malmer B, Henriksson R, Gronberg H: Familial brain tumours – genetics or environment? A nationwide cohort study of cancer risk in spouses and first-degree relatives of brain tumour patients. Int J Cancer 2003;106:260–263.
26 Malmer B, Iselius L, Holmberg E, Collins A, Henriksson R, Gronberg H: Genetic epidemiology of glioma. Br J Cancer 2001;84:429–434.
27 Schlehofer B, Blettner M, Becker N, Martinsohn C, Wahrendorf J: Medical risk factors and the development of brain tumors. Cancer 1992;69:2541–2547.
28 Wrensch MR, Barger GR: Familial factors associated with malignant gliomas. Genet Epidemiol 1990;7:291–301.
29 Zampieri P, Meneghini F, Grigoletto F, Gerosa M, Licata C, Casentini L, Longatti PL, Padoan A, Mingrino S: Risk factors for cerebral glioma in adults: a case-control study in an Italian population. J Neurooncol 1994;19:61–67.
30 Malmer B, Henriksson R, Gronberg H: Different aetiology of familial low-grade and high-grade glioma? A nationwide cohort study of familial glioma. Neuroepidemiology 2002;21:279–286.
31 de Andrade M, Barnholtz JS, Amos CI, Adatto P, Spencer C, Bondy ML: Segregation analysis of cancer in families of glioma patients. Genet Epidemiol 2001;20:258–270.
32 Grossman SA, Osman M, Hruban R, Piantadosi S: Central nervous system cancers in first-degree relatives and spouses. Cancer Invest 1999;17:299–308.
33 Elexpuru-Camiruaga J, Buxton N, Kandula V, Dias PS, Campbell D, McIntosh J, Broome J, Jones P, Inskip A, Alldersea J: Susceptibility to astrocytoma and meningioma: influence of allelism at glutathione S-transferase (GSTT1 and GSTM1) and cytochrome P-450 (CYP2D6) loci. Cancer Res 1995;55:4237–4239.
34 Kelsey KT, Wrensch M, Zuo ZF, Miike R, Wiencke JK: A population-based case-control study of the CYP2D6 and GSTT1 polymorphisms and malignant brain tumors. Pharmacogenetics 1997;7:463–468.
35 Trizna Z, de Andrade M, Kyritsis AP, Briggs K, Levin VA, Bruner JM, Wei Q, Bondy ML: Genetic polymorphisms in glutathione S-transferase mu and theta, N-acetyltransferase, and CYP1A1 and risk of gliomas. Cancer Epidemiol Biomarkers Prev 1998;7:553–555.
36 De Roos AJ, Rothman N, Inskip PD, Linet MS, Shapiro WR, Selker RG, Fine HA, Black PM, Pittman GS, Bell DA: Genetic polymorphisms in GSTM1, -P1, -T1, and CYP2E1 and the risk of adult brain tumors. Cancer Epidemiol Biomarkers Prev 2003;12:14–22.
37 Hand PA, Inskip A, Gilford J, Alldersea J, Elexpuru-Camiruaga J, Hayes JD, Jones PW, Strange RC, Fryer AA: Allelism at the glutathione S-transferase GSTM3 locus: interactions with GSTM1 and GSTT1 as risk factors for astrocytoma. Carcinogenesis 1996;17:1919–1922.
38 Wrensch M, Kelsey KT, Liu M, Miike R, Moghadassi M, Aldape K, McMillan A, Wiencke J: Glutathione-S-transferase and adult glioma. Cancer Epidemiol Biomarkers Prev 2004;13: 461–467.
39 Chen P, Wiencke J, Aldape K, Kesler-Diaz A, Miike R, Kelsey K, Lee M, Liu J, Wrensch M: Association of an ERCC1 polymorphism with adult-onset glioma. Cancer Epidemiol Biomarkers Prev 2000;9:843–847.
40 Caggana M, Kilgallen J, Conroy JM, Wiencke JK, Kelsey KT, Miike R, Chen P, Wrensch MR: Associations between ERCC2 polymorphisms and gliomas. Cancer Epidemiol Biomarkers Prev 2001;10:355–360.
41 Wacholder S, Chanock S, Garcia-Closas M, El Ghormli L, Rothman N: Assessing the probability that a positive report is false: an approach for molecular epidemiology studies. J Natl Cancer Inst 2004;96:434–442.
42 Bondy ML, Kyritsis AP, Gu J, de Andrade M, Cunningham J, Levin VA, Bruner JM, Wei Q: Mutagen sensitivity and risk of gliomas: a case-control analysis. Cancer Res 1996;56:1484–1486.

43 Nersesyan AK: Re: Gamma-radiation sensitivity and risk of glioma. J Natl Cancer Inst 2002; 94:949.
44 Fisher SG, Weber L, Carbone M: Cancer risk associated with simian virus 40 contaminated polio vaccine. Anticancer Res 1999;19:2173–2180.
45 Geissler E, Staneczek W: SV40 and human brain tumors. Arch Geschwulstforsch 1988;58: 129–134.
46 Strickler HD, Rosenberg PS, Devesa SS, Hertel J, Fraumeni JFJ, Goedert JJ: Contamination of poliovirus vaccines with simian virus 40 (1955–1963) and subsequent cancer rates. JAMA 1998;279:292–295.
47 Wrensch M, Weinberg A, Wiencke J, Masters H, Miike R, Barger G, Lee M: Does prior infection with varicella-zoster virus influence risk of adult glioma? Am J Epidemiol 1997;145:594–597.
48 Wrensch M, Weinberg A, Wiencke J, Miike R, Barger G, Kelsey K: Prevalence of antibodies to four herpesviruses among adults with glioma and controls. Am J Epidemiol 2001;154:161–165.
49 Caldarelli-Stefano R, Boldorini R, Monga G, Meraviglia E, Zorini EO, Ferrante P: JC virus in human glial-derived tumors. Hum Pathol 2000;31:394–395.
50 Croul S, Otte J, Khalili K: Brain tumors and polyomaviruses. J Neurovirol 2003;9:173–182.
51 Del Valle L, Gordon J, Assimakopoulou M, Enam S, Geddes JF, Varakis JN, Katsetos CD, Croul S, Khalili K: Detection of JC virus DNA sequences and expression of the viral regulatory protein T-antigen in tumors of the central nervous system. Cancer Res 2001;61:4287–4293.
52 Dorries K, Loeber G, Meixensberger J: Association of polyomaviruses JC, SV40, and BK with human brain tumors. Virology 1987;160:268–270.
53 Krynska B, Otte J, Franks R, Khalili K, Croul S: Human ubiquitous JCV(CY) T-antigen gene induces brain tumors in experimental animals. Oncogene 1999;18:39–46.
54 Tretiakova A, Krynska B, Gordon J, Khalili K: Human neurotropic JC virus early protein deregulates glial cell cycle pathway and impairs cell differentiation. J Neurosci Res 1999;55:588–599.
55 Cuomo L, Trivedi P, Cardillo MR, Gagliardi FM, Vecchione A, Caruso R, Calogero A, Frati L, Faggioni A, Ragona G: Human herpesvirus 6 infection in neoplastic and normal brain tissue. J Med Virol 2001;63:45–51.
56 Rollison DEM, Helzlsouer KJ, Alberg AJ, Hoffman S, Hou J, Daniel R, Shah KV, Major EO: Serum antibodies to JC virus, BK virus, simian virus 40, and the risk of incident adult astrocytic brain tumors. Cancer Epidemiol Biomarkers Prev 2003;12:460–463.
57 Blumenthal DT, Raizer JJ, Rosenblum MK, Bilsky MH, Hariharan S, Abrey LE: Primary intracranial neoplasms in patients with HIV. Neurology 1999;52:1648–1651.
58 Fisher J, Schwartzbaum J, Johnson C: Cold/influenza infection, influenza vaccination, and risk of adult glioma (abstract). Am J Epidemiol 2000;151:116.
59 Schlehofer B, Blettner M, Preston-Martin S, Niehoff D, Wahrendorf J, Arslan A, Ahlbom A, Choi WN, Giles GG, Howe GR, Little J, Menegoz F, Ryan P: Role of medical history in brain tumour development. Results from the international adult brain tumour study. Int J Cancer 1999;82: 155–160.
60 Ryan P, Hurley SF, Johnson AM, Salzberg M, Lee MW, North JB, McNeil JJ, McMichael AJ: Tumours of the brain and presence of antibodies to *Toxoplasma gondii*. Int J Epidemiol 1993;22: 412–419.
61 Schuman LM, Choi NW, Gullen WH: Relationship of central nervous system neoplasms to *Toxoplasma gondii* infection. Am J Publ Health Nations Health 1967;57:848–856.
62 Brenner AV, Linet MS, Fine HA, Shapiro WR, Selker RG, Black PM, Inskip PD: History of allergies and autoimmune diseases and risk of brain tumors in adults. Int J Cancer 2002;99: 252–259.
63 Schwartzbaum J, Jonsson F, Ahlbom A, Preston-Martin S, Lonn S, Soderberg KC, Feychting M: Cohort studies of association between self-reported allergic conditions, immune-related diagnoses and glioma and meningioma risk. Int J Cancer 2003;106:423–428.
64 Venge P: Monitoring the allergic inflammation. Allergy 2004;59:26–32.
65 Wiemels JL, Wiencke JK, Sison JD, Miike R, McMillan A, Wrensch M: History of allergies among adults with glioma and controls. Int J Cancer 2002;98:609–615.
66 Ryan P, Lee MW, North B, McMichael AJ: Risk factors for tumors of the brain and meninges: results from the Adelaide Adult Brain Tumor Study. Int J Cancer 1992;51:20–27.

67 Phillips LE, Koepsell TD, van Belle G, Kukull WA, Gehrels J-A, Longstreth WTJ: History of head trauma and risk of intracranial meningioma: population-based case-control study. Neurology 2002;58:1849–1852.

68 Preston-Martin S, Mack W, Henderson BE: Risk factors for gliomas and meningiomas in males in Los Angeles County. Cancer Res 1989;49:6137–6143.

69 Preston-Martin S, Pogoda JM, Schlehofer B, Blettner M, Howe GR, Ryan P, Menegoz F, Giles GG, Rodvall Y, Choi NW, Little J, Arslan A: An international case-control study of adult glioma and meningioma: the role of head trauma. Int J Epidemiol 1998;27:579–586.

70 Preston-Martin S, Yu MC, Henderson BE, Roberts C: Risk factors for meningiomas in men in Los Angeles County. J Natl Cancer Inst 1983;70:863–866.

71 Annegers JF, Laws ERJ, Kurland LT, Grabow JD: Head trauma and subsequent brain tumors. Neurosurgery 1979;4:203–236.

72 Inskip PD, Mellemkjaer L, Gridley G, Olsen JH: Incidence of intracranial tumors following hospitalization for head injuries (Denmark). Cancer Causes Control 1998;9:109–116.

73 Nygren C, Adami J, Ye W, Bellocco R, af Geijerstam JL, Borg J, Nyren O: Primary brain tumors following traumatic brain injury – a population-based cohort study in Sweden. Cancer Causes Control 2001;12:733–737.

74 Hu J, Johnson KC, Mao Y, Guo L, Zhao X, Jia X, Bi D, Huang G, Liu R: Risk factors for glioma in adults: a case-control study in northeast China. Cancer Detect Prev 1998;22:100–108.

75 Hochberg F, Toniolo P, Cole P: Head trauma and seizures as risk factors of glioblastoma. Neurology 1984;34:1511–1514.

76 Wrensch M, Miike R, Lee M, Neuhaus J: Are prior head injuries or diagnostic X-rays associated with glioma in adults? The effects of control selection bias. Neuroepidemiology 2000;19: 234–244.

77 Pace A, Bove L, Innocenti P, Pietrangeli A, Carapella CM, Oppido P, Raus L, Occhipinti E, Jandolo B: Epilepsy and gliomas: incidence and treatment in 119 patients. J Exp Clin Cancer Res 1998;17:479–482.

78 Lamminpaa A, Pukkala E, Teppo L, Neuvonen PJ: Cancer incidence among patients using antiepileptic drugs: a long-term follow-up of 28,000 patients. Eur J Clin Pharmacol 2002;58: 137–141.

79 Schwartzbaum J, Jonsson F, Ahlbom A, Preston-Martin S, Malmer B, Lonn S, Soderberg KC, Feychting M: Prior hospitalization for epilepsy, diabetes, and stroke may result from preclinical systemic effects of astrocytoma and meningioma. Submitted.

80 Olsen JH, Boice JDJ, Jensen JP, Fraumeni JFJ: Cancer among epileptic patients exposed to anticonvulsant drugs. J Natl Cancer Inst 1989;81:803–808.

81 Shirts SB, Annegers JF, Hauser WA, Kurland LT: Cancer incidence in a cohort of patients with seizure disorders. J Natl Cancer Inst 1986;77:83–87.

82 Bondy M, Ligon BL: Epidemiology and etiology of intracranial meningiomas: a review. J Neurooncol 1996;29:197–205.

83 Longstreth WTJ, Dennis LK, McGuire VM, Drangsholt MT, Koepsell TD: Epidemiology of intracranial meningioma. Cancer 1993;72:639–648.

84 Horsfall DJ, Goldsmith KG, Ricciardelli C, Skinner JM, Tilley WD, Marshall VR: Steroid hormone and epidermal growth factor receptors in meningiomas. Aust NZ J Surg 1989;59:881–888.

85 Punnonen R, Kuurne T: Estrogen and progestin receptors in intracranial tumors. Horm Res 1987;27:74–77.

86 Yu ZY, Wrange O, Haglund B, Granholm L, Gustafsson JA: Estrogen and progestin receptors in intracranial meningiomas. J Steroid Biochem 1982;16:451–456.

87 Jhawar BS, Fuchs CS, Colditz GA, Stampfer MJ: Sex steroid hormone exposures and risk for meningioma. J Neurosurg 2003;99:848–853.

88 Schlehofer B, Blettner M, Wahrendorf J: Association between brain tumors and menopausal status. J Natl Cancer Inst 1992;84:1346–1349.

89 Lambe M, Coogan P, Baron J: Reproductive factors and the risk of brain tumors: a population-based study in Sweden. Int J Cancer 1997;72:389–393.

90 McKinley BP, Michalek AM, Fenstermaker RA, Plunkett RJ: The impact of age and sex on the incidence of glial tumors in New York state from 1976 to 1995. J Neurosurg 2000;93:932–939.

91 Cantor KP, Lynch CF, Johnson D: Reproductive factors and risk of brain, colon, and other malignancies in Iowa (United States). Cancer Causes Control 1993;4:505–511.
92 Preston-Martin S, Henderson BE: N-Nitroso compounds and human intracranial tumours. IARC Sci Publ 1984;57:887–894.
93 Chen H, Ward MH, Tucker KL, Graubard BI, McComb RD, Potischman NA, Weisenburger DD, Heineman EF: Diet and risk of adult glioma in eastern Nebraska, United States. Cancer Causes Control 2002;13:647–655.
94 Lee M, Wrensch M, Miike R: Dietary and tobacco risk factors for adult onset glioma in the San Francisco Bay Area (California, USA). Cancer Causes Control 1997;8:13–24.
95 Schwartzbaum JA, Fisher JL, Goodman J, Octaviano D, Cornwell DG: Hypotheses concerning roles of dietary energy, cured meat, and serum tocopherols in adult glioma development. Neuroepidemiology 1999;18:156–166.
96 Huncharek M, Kupelnick B, Wheeler L: Dietary cured meat and the risk of adult glioma: a meta-analysis of nine observational studies. J Environ Pathol Toxicol Oncol 2003;22:129–137.
97 Barrett JH, Parslow RC, McKinney PA, Law GR, Forman D: Nitrate in drinking water and the incidence of gastric, esophageal, and brain cancer in Yorkshire, England. Cancer Causes Control 1998;9:153–159.
98 Hu J, La Vecchia C, Negri E, Chatenoud L, Bosetti C, Jia X, Liu R, Huang G, Bi D, Wang C: Diet and brain cancer in adults: a case-control study in northeast China. Int J Cancer 1999;81:20–23.
99 Tedeschi-Blok N, Schwartzbaum J, Lee M, Miike R, Wrensch M: Dietary calcium consumption and astrocytic glioma: the San Francisco Bay Area Adult Glioma Study, 1991–1995. Nutr Cancer 2001;39:196–203.
100 Hurley SF, McNeil JJ, Donnan GA, Forbes A, Salzberg M, Giles GG: Tobacco smoking and alcohol consumption as risk factors for glioma: a case-control study in Melbourne, Australia. J Epidemiol Community Health 1996;50:442–446.
101 Hu J, Little J, Xu T, Zhao X, Guo L, Jia X, Huang G, Bi D, Liu R: Risk factors for meningioma in adults: a case-control study in northeast China. Int J Cancer 1999;83:299–304.
102 Preston-Martin S, Mack W: Gliomas and meningiomas in men in Los Angeles County: investigation of exposures to N-nitroso compounds. IARC Sci Publ 1991;105:197–203.
103 Grayson JK, Lyons TJ: Brain cancer, flying, and socioeconomic status: a nested case-control study of USAF aircrew. Aviat Space Environ Med 1996;67:1152–1154.
104 Gundestrup M, Storm HH: Radiation-induced acute myeloid leukaemia and other cancers in commercial jet cockpit crew: a population-based cohort study. Lancet 1999;354:2029–2031.
105 Alexander V, DiMarco JH: Reappraisal of brain tumor risk among U.S. nuclear workers: a 10-year review. Occup Med 2001;16:289–315.
106 Loomis DP, Wolf SH: Mortality of workers at a nuclear materials production plant at Oak Ridge, Tennessee, 1947–1990. Am J Ind Med 1996;29:131–141.
107 Hardell L, Mild KH, Pahlson A, Hallquist A: Ionizing radiation, cellular telephones and the risk for brain tumours. Eur J Cancer Prev 2001;10:523–529.
108 Hodges LC, Smith JL, Garrett A, Tate S: Prevalence of glioblastoma multiforme in subjects with prior therapeutic radiation. J Neurosci Nurs 1992;24:79–83.
109 Salvati M, Artico M, Caruso R, Rocchi G, Orlando ER, Nucci F: A report on radiation-induced gliomas. Cancer 1991;67:392–397.
110 Shapiro S, Mealey JJ, Sartorius C: Radiation-induced intracranial malignant gliomas. J Neurosurg 1989;71:77–82.
111 Salminen E, Pukkala E, Teppo L: Second cancers in patients with brain tumours – impact of treatment. Eur J Cancer 1999;35:102–105.
112 Longstreth WTJ, Phillips LE, Drangsholt M, Koepsell TD, Custer BS, Gehrels J-A, van Belle G: Dental X-rays and the risk of intracranial meningioma: a population-based case-control study. Cancer 2004;100:1026–1034.
113 Shintani T, Hayakawa N, Hoshi M, Sumida M, Kurisu K, Oki S, Kodama Y, Kajikawa H, Inai K, Kamada N: High incidence of meningioma among Hiroshima atomic bomb survivors. J Radiat Res 1999;40:49–57.
114 Rothman KJ, Loughlin JE, Funch DP, Dreyer NA: Overall mortality of cellular telephone customers. Epidemiology 1996;7:303–305.

115 Auvinen A, Hietanen M, Luukkonen R, Koskela R-S: Brain tumors and salivary gland cancers among cellular telephone users. Epidemiology 2002;13:356–359.
116 Hardell L, Nasman A, Pahlson A, Hallquist A, Hansson Mild K: Use of cellular telephones and the risk for brain tumours: a case-control study. Int J Oncol 1999;15:113–116.
117 Inskip PD, Tarone RE, Hatch EE, Wilcosky TC, Shapiro WR, Selker RG, Fine HA, Black PM, Loeffler JS, Linet MS: Cellular-telephone use and brain tumors. N Engl J Med 2001;344:79–86.
118 Muscat JE, Malkin MG, Thompson S, Shore RE, Stellman SD, McRee D, Neugut AI, Wynder EL: Handheld cellular telephone use and risk of brain cancer. JAMA 2000;284:3001–3007.
119 Johansen C, Boice JJ, McLaughlin J, Olsen J: Cellular telephones and cancer – a nationwide cohort study in Denmark. J Natl Cancer Inst 2001;93:203–207.
120 Hardell L, Mild KH, Carlberg M: Case-control study on the use of cellular and cordless phones and the risk for malignant brain tumours. Int J Radiat Biol 2002;78:931–936.
121 Hardell L, Mild KH, Carlberg M: Further aspects on cellular and cordless telephones and brain tumours. Int J Oncol 2003;22:399–407.
122 De Roos AJ, Stewart PA, Linet MS, Heineman EF, Dosemeci M, Wilcosky T, Shapiro WR, Selker RG, Fine HA, Black PM, Inskip PD: Occupation and the risk of adult glioma in the United States. Cancer Causes Control 2003;14:139–150.
123 Floderus B, Persson T, Stenlund C, Wennberg A, Ost A, Knave B: Occupational exposure to electromagnetic fields in relation to leukemia and brain tumors: a case-control study in Sweden. Cancer Causes Control 1993;4:465–476.
124 Floderus B, Stenlund C, Persson T: Occupational magnetic field exposure and site-specific cancer incidence: a Swedish cohort study. Cancer Causes Control 1999;10:323–332.
125 Lin RS, Dischinger PC, Conde J, Farrell KP: Occupational exposure to electromagnetic fields and the occurrence of brain tumors. An analysis of possible associations. J Occup Med 1985;27: 413–419.
126 Mack W, Preston-Martin S, Peters JM: Astrocytoma risk related to job exposure to electric and magnetic fields. Bioelectromagnetics 1991;12:57–66.
127 Preston-Martin S, Lewis S, Winkelmann R, Borman B, Auld J, Pearce N: Descriptive epidemiology of primary cancer of the brain, cranial nerves, and cranial meninges in New Zealand, 1948–88. Cancer Causes Control 1993;4:529–538.
128 Rodvall Y, Ahlbom A, Stenlund C, Preston-Martin S, Lindh T, Spannare B: Occupational exposure to magnetic fields and brain tumours in central Sweden. Eur J Epidemiol 1998;14:563–569.
129 Speers MA, Dobbins JG, Miller VS: Occupational exposures and brain cancer mortality: a preliminary study of east Texas residents. Am J Ind Med 1988;13:629–638.
130 Spinelli JJ, Band PR, Svirchev LM, Gallagher RP: Mortality and cancer incidence in aluminum reduction plant workers. J Occup Med 1991;33:1150–1155.
131 Villeneuve PJ, Agnew DA, Johnson KC, Mao Y: Brain cancer and occupational exposure to magnetic fields among men: results from a Canadian population-based case-control study. Int J Epidemiol 2002;31:210–217.
132 Zheng T, Cantor KP, Zhang Y, Keim S, Lynch CF: Occupational risk factors for brain cancer: a population-based case-control study in Iowa. J Occup Environ Med 2001;43:317–324.
133 Johansen C, Olsen JH: Risk of cancer among Danish electricity workers. A cohort study. Ugeskr Laeger 1999;161:2079–2085.
134 Minder CE, Pfluger DH: Leukemia, brain tumors, and exposure to extremely low frequency electromagnetic fields in Swiss railway employees. Am J Epidemiol 2001;153:825–835.
135 Sahl JD, Kelsh MA, Greenland S: Cohort and nested case-control studies of hematopoietic cancers and brain cancer among electric utility workers. Epidemiology 1993;4:104–114.
136 Sorahan T, Nichols L, van Tongeren M, Harrington JM: Occupational exposure to magnetic fields relative to mortality from brain tumours: updated and revised findings from a study of United Kingdom electricity generation and transmission workers, 1973–97. Occup Environ Med 2001;58: 626–630.
137 Tynes T, Jynge H, Vistnes AI: Leukemia and brain tumors in Norwegian railway workers, a nested case-control study. Am J Epidemiol 1994;139:645–653.
138 Fear NT, Roman E, Carpenter LM, Newton R, Bull D: Cancer in electrical workers: an analysis of cancer registrations in England, 1981–87. Br J Cancer 1996;73:935–939.

139 Grayson JK: Radiation exposure, socioeconomic status, and brain tumor risk in the US Air Force: a nested case-control study. Am J Epidemiol 1996;143:480–486.
140 Navas-Acien A, Pollan M, Gustavsson P, Floderus B, Plato N, Dosemeci M: Interactive effect of chemical substances and occupational electromagnetic field exposure on the risk of gliomas and meningiomas in Swedish men. Cancer Epidemiol Biomarkers Prev 2002;11:1678–1683.
141 Savitz DA, Cai J, van Wijngaarden E, Loomis D, Mihlan G, Dufort V, Kleckner RC, Nylander-French L, Kromhout H, Zhou H: Case-cohort analysis of brain cancer and leukemia in electric utility workers using a refined magnetic field job-exposure matrix. Am J Ind Med 2000;38:417–425.
142 Wrensch M, Yost M, Miike R, Lee G, Touchstone J: Adult glioma in relation to residential power frequency electromagnetic field exposures in the San Francisco Bay area. Epidemiology 1999;10: 523–527.

James L. Fisher, PhD
The Arthur G. James Cancer Hospital and Richard J. Solove Research Institute
2050 Kenny Road Suite 940
Columbus, OH 43221 (USA)
Tel. +1 614 293 9644, Fax +1 614 293 6667, E-Mail jay.fisher@osumc.edu

Pollock BE (ed): Guiding Neurosurgery by Evidence.
Prog Neurol Surg. Basel, Karger, 2006, vol 19, pp 80–96

Benign Adult Brain Tumors: An Evidence-Based Medicine Review

Manish Aghi, Fred G. Barker II

Neurosurgical Service, Massachusetts General Hospital, Boston, Mass., USA

Abstract

Background: Benign adult brain tumors can be managed conservatively or using surgery, radiation, or medicines. While randomized comparisons assessing tumor recurrence, quality of life, or survival are the ideal means of comparing treatments, it can be difficult to recruit patients to such trials and lengthy follow-up periods are needed because of the slowly progressive natural history of these tumors. **Methods:** Review of the literature on benign adult brain tumors using evidence-based standards and focusing on meningiomas, pituitary adenomas, and vestibular schwannomas, which together represent the majority of WHO grade 1 adult brain tumors. **Results:** Nearly all studies of benign adult brain tumors were of relatively poor quality (level 3 or poorer). These studies enable grade C recommendations. The safety of meningioma surgery in the elderly varies with institution, radiosurgery is a reliable alternative to surgery in small to medium-sized meningiomas, and the efficacy of drugs in therapy of meningiomas recurring after surgery is difficult to interpret due to a lack of uniform criteria in the studies. Radiosurgery is effective in nonfunctional pituitary adenomas recurring after surgery, while phototherapy is a newer treatment modality with potential benefits in pituitary adenomas that fail surgery or radiation. Vestibular schwannomas can be conservatively managed, but there are no reliable predictors of growth, so serial imaging is important. Radiosurgery has proven to be a reliable alternative to surgery for small to medium-sized vestibular schwannomas, but follow-up has been relatively short in most studies to date. **Conclusions:** While randomized clinical trials comparing conservative management, surgery, radiation, and medical management of benign adult benign tumors are unlikely to occur, there is some level 3 evidence that can assist in their treatment.

Each year, slightly more than 40,000 individuals in the United States are diagnosed with brain tumors [1]. Of these, 43% are benign brain tumors [1], although an accurate accounting is difficult to obtain because most state cancer registries historically have collected data only on primary malignant brain tumors. Benign adult brain tumors comprise both intra-axial and extra-axial tumors and include epidermoid, dermoid, hemangioblastoma, colloid cyst, subependymoma, pleomorphic xanthoastrocytoma, schwannoma, pituitary adenoma, craniopharyngioma and meningioma. Here we review the literature for treatment studies on meningiomas, pituitary adenomas, and vestibular schwannomas using evidence-based standards. Because these three neoplasms collectively account for 40% of all intracranial neoplasms [2–4], they have generated enough studies on treatment options that some recommendations can be made based on evidence-based standards. Unfortunately the paucity of randomized clinical trials in this field leads to an inability to make high grade recommendations. In addition, with benign tumors, the success of a treatment in preventing recurrence or progression may not be evident for 10 or more years after surgery. Thus, information derived from case series (level 4 evidence) or case-control (level 3 evidence) studies is often the best available data on which to base clinical decisions for patients with benign brain tumors. Despite these constraints, the studies described in this chapter provide some important insight into treatment options for these three common benign brain tumors.

Meningiomas

Meningiomas represent approximately 15% of adult intracranial neoplasms [3]. Up to one third of meningiomas diagnosed during life are asymptomatic [5], a number that will likely grow as imaging technologies improve and the use of cranial imaging in patients with minimal symptoms increases. As a result, a common challenge facing the neurosurgeon is the advisability of surgical resection of asymptomatic meningiomas. Level 3 evidence addressing this issue came from a retrospective record review identifying 504 meningiomas diagnosed at 27 hospitals in a region of Japan between 1989 and 1996 [6]. Of these meningiomas, 39% were asymptomatic, a proportion that was increasing over time. Asymptomatic meningiomas were more common in older patients and female patients. Surgery was performed on 87 of 196 asymptomatic meningiomas. In 20 of the 63 conservatively managed meningiomas, the tumor increased in size during the follow-up period. The tendency to increase in size did not depend on initial size, age, or gender; T2 bright tumors were more likely to grow; and calcified tumors were less likely to grow during follow-up. Morbidity occurred in 11.4% of asymptomatic patients who underwent surgery, including 23.3% of patients older than 70 years, compared to 3.5% of patients younger than 70. The study did not support surgery in elderly patients with asymptomatic meningiomas.

Surgical resection has long been the preferred treatment modality for symptomatic meningiomas. In 1957, Simpson [7] published a landmark paper documenting the direct correlation between degree of meningioma resection and later tumor recurrence. He reported a 9% recurrence rate after 'complete resection' of the tumor and its neoplastic dural base (grade 1 resection), a 19% recurrence rate when the tumor was resected and the dural base only coagulated (grade 2), a 29% recurrence rate when the tumor itself was removed but the dura could not be excised (grade 3), and an approximately 40% recurrence rate when only subtotal resection was performed (grade 4). Simpson's recurrence rates may have been an underestimate, because his study preceded the availability of CT or MRI. Subsequent studies found a 70% rate of tumor progression after subtotal resection alone [8], and 16 and 20% recurrence rates after grade 1 and 2 resections [9]. Given this recurrence rate after grade 1 resections, in 1986 Borovich and colleagues [10, 11] recommended adding another grade, 'grade 0', defined by an excision in which a 2-cm-wide resection of normal dural margin occurred. In a subsequent level 4 study, a retrospective review of grade 0 removal of convexity meningiomas in 37 patients between 1982 and 1992 at three different centers found no recurrences and no increase in morbidity with the more aggressive procedure [12]. Of course, comparisons to other studies describing grade 1 resections cannot be made because those series may have contained a mix of grade 0 and grade 1 resections.

Many meningiomas occur in older persons, with a peak incidence at 60 years [13]. Because surgery often carries an elevated level of risk in elderly patients, surgeons need evidence to determine the role of age in deciding whether to resect a meningioma. In a case-control study, a prospectively acquired database was used to identify 114 patients undergoing meningioma resection by a single surgeon [14]. The patients were divided into those 65 and over and those under 65, with each group having 57 patients. More than 90% of the meningiomas in each group were symptomatic. Medical and surgical complication rates were 7.0 and 5.2% in elderly patients, compared to 8.8 and 3.5% in younger patients ($p > 0.05$). Mortality within the first 30 postoperative days was zero for the younger patients, and 1/57 in the older group ($p > 0.05$). This study provided level 3 evidence confirming the safety of meningioma surgery in elderly patients. Of note, significantly less morbidity was found in this study than in previous studies of meningioma surgery in the elderly [14], suggesting that the advisability of meningioma surgery in the elderly may vary from center to center.

More recently, stereotactic radiosurgery has been used as an alternative to surgical excision for some patients with small- to moderate-sized meningiomas. There has been only one study comparing the efficacy of radiosurgery to that of surgical resection for intracranial meningiomas. A retrospective cohort design was used to compare outcomes between 528 patients who underwent surgical resection versus 170 patients who underwent radiosurgery for intracranial meningiomas from 1990 to 1997 at the Mayo Clinic [15]. While surgery patients were retrospectively identified, information on radiosurgery patients was retrieved from a prospectively maintained computer database. Tumor recurrence or progression occurred in 12% of patients in the surgical resection group, more frequently than the 2% rate in the radiosurgery group ($p = 0.05$). The 3- and 7-year actuarial progression free survival for patients having Simpson Grade 1 surgical resections were 100 and 96%, comparable to the 100 and 95% obtained with radiosurgery ($p = 0.94$). On the other hand, Simpson Grade 2 resections produced 91 and 82% 3- and 7-year progression-free survivals, less than obtained with radiosurgery ($p < 0.05$). This study provides level 3 evidence supporting radiosurgery in the management of patients with small- to moderate-sized meningiomas without symptomatic mass effect, especially those for which an incomplete resection is anticipated.

Other studies have focused on medical treatment of unresectable or recurrent meningiomas, but are difficult to interpret because of varying endpoints used and varying duration of follow-up. Because 70% of meningiomas express the progesterone receptor and meningiomas grow more rapidly when exposed to progesterone during pregnancy, antiprogesterone agents have been investigated in the treatment of unresectable meningiomas. One of these antiprogesterone agents, mifepristone, was studied in one of the few randomized trials in benign brain tumors. Results of a phase III randomized placebo-controlled study of mifepristone for unresectable histologically confirmed meningioma which had appeared or progressed within 2 years were presented in 2001 [16]. Eighty patients received mifepristone, and 80 received placebo. The two groups were comparable in age, gender, and use of prior radiation. Progression was defined as anatomic growth or neurologic deterioration. There was no significant difference in response, with a median time to progression of 10 months with mifepristone and 12 months with placebo ($p = 0.44$).

Interferon-α, a putative angiostatic agent, was studied in 11 patients with postoperative residual meningioma [17]. In this study, the endpoint was average percentage change in the methionine uptake ratio on positron emission tomography (PET) per patient over serial PET exams taken every 2–4 weeks after initiating treatment, with a mean of 5.4 PET studies per patient over a mean observation period of 2 years. Nine of 12 patients were responders, defined as experiencing a reduction in methionine uptake. The responders averaged 30.4% reduction in methionine uptake. The 3 nonresponders averaged a 1.8% increase in methionine uptake. While this study represents the only one cited here in which a medical agent proved beneficial in meningioma therapy, the lack of a control group and the unique reliance on PET scan data rather than the more commonly used MRI volume make data from this study difficult to interpret.

A prospective phase II study of temozolomide for treatment-resistant recurrent meningioma enrolled 16 patients with meningiomas that had recurred after surgery and progressed following radiotherapy [18]. Patients received 10-week cycles of temozolomide. No patient demonstrated a neuroradiographic complete or partial response, defined by volume on MRI. Time to tumor progression ranged from 2.5 to 5.0 months; survival ranged from 4 to 9 months. As a result, this level 4 study was terminated following the enrollment of the first 16 patients. Given the poor survival in this group and the limitation to patients whose tumors progressed following radiotherapy, these patients may represent a subset of WHO grade I meningiomas with a particularly poor prognosis compared to the patients included in other studies. A phase II clinical trial in the United States sponsored by the Southwest Oncology Group with principal investigators at Johns Hopkins is underway to study hydroxyurea in treating up to 38 patients with recurrent or histologically confirmed unresectable benign meningioma who experienced disease progression after radiotherapy [19].

Pituitary Adenomas

Pituitary adenomas account for 10–15% of intracranial neoplasms, placing them third in frequency behind gliomas and meningiomas [2]. Transsphenoidal resection has been the mainstay of pituitary adenoma treatment since it was first reported in 1907 by Schloffer [20]. Over the last 20 years, medicine has replaced surgery as initial treatment for nearly half of the pituitary adenomas that secrete prolactin. In 1985, a prospective multicenter trial investigated the effects of dopamine agonist bromocriptine in reducing the size of prolactin-secreting macroadenomas with extrasellar extension [21]. Prolactin levels were normalized in 18 of 27 patients. In 13 patients (46%), tumor size was reduced by greater than 50%, in 5 patients (18%) by about 50%, and in 9 patients (36%) by 10–25%. In this series, in the 4 patients in whom bromocriptine was stopped after 1 year, tumor regrowth occurred in 3 patients. Treatment was well tolerated. In the long term, only about 20% of patients can stop bromocriptine and maintain normal prolactin levels [22]. Between 5 and 10% of patients with prolactinomas do not respond to bromocriptine [23]. Although not compared by a randomized trial, results with bromocriptine treatment compare favorably to results with transsphenoidal surgery. A summary of surgical results from 34 published series shows that 73.7% of microadenomas and 32.4% of macroadenomas were reported to have normal prolactin levels 1–12 weeks following surgery [24]. As a result, prolactin testing and bromocriptine therapy of prolactinomas have become standard before attempting surgical resection of pituitary masses except in unusual circumstances.

Nearly one fourth of pituitary adenomas are nonfunctional tumors [25]. In one retrospective study, patients with nonfunctioning pituitary adenomas treated between 1961 and 1996 at a single institution were analyzed to compare the response to radiation alone in 38 patients versus surgery followed by radiation in 97 patients [26]. Recurrence, tumor progression, and postoperative hypopituitarism did not differ between the two groups. This study concluded that nonfunctioning pituitary adenomas could be safely treated with radiation alone, especially for patients unable to tolerate surgery.

Because they fail to develop symptoms from tumor hormone secretion when their tumors are still small, patients with nonfunctional adenomas present with larger tumors that are more likely to exhibit dural invasion, leading to reported postoperative radiographic recurrence rates ranging from 23 to 46% [27, 28]. The management of patients with nonfunctioning adenomas that undergo incomplete surgical removal was investigated in a study in which 119 patients with residual or recurrent postoperative adenoma after surgery at a single institution were retrospectively reviewed [29]. There were 68 patients who did not undergo adjunctive radiation, and 51 patients who underwent gamma knife surgery within 1 year of surgery. Regrowth of residual tumor occurred in 47.1% of nonradiated and 3.9% of radiated patients ($p < 0.001$). This led to level 3 evidence supporting gamma knife treatment for incompletely removed nonfunctional pituitary adenomas. While the two groups were balanced with respect to demographics, tumor size prior to surgery, and duration of follow-up, tumor size after surgery was not stated.

Hormonally active pituitary adenomas that are incompletely resected are a concern even when they do not undergo growth of the residual tumor, because of the dangers posed by continuing excess hormone secretion. This is particularly true for patients with acromegaly, because untreated acromegaly leads to illness and premature death due to heart disease and possibly development of malignant tumors [30]. One group compared the results of radiosurgery to fractionated radiation therapy for patients with recurrent acromegaly after surgery [31]. Using a retrospective review of records at a Swiss center, 50 patients who underwent fractionated radiation (median dose 40 Gy) from 1973 to 1992 were compared to 16 patients having radiosurgery (median tumor margin dose 25 Gy) between 1994 and 1996 [31]. The radiation therapy group was followed for considerably longer, but the groups were otherwise similar with regard to demographics, tumor size, and pretreatment levels of growth hormone and insulin-like growth factor I. Patients having radiosurgery more commonly achieved biochemical remission ($p < 0.0001$); the mean time to endocrine normalization was 1.4 years after radiosurgery compared to 7.1 years after fractionated radiation therapy. This study provided level 3 evidence in favor of radiosurgery over fractionated radiation for patients with recurrent acromegaly.

The possibility of reducing the incidence of incomplete surgical removal of pituitary adenomas by using intraoperative MRI was investigated in 39 patients with pituitary macroadenomas treated at the University of Cincinnati between 1998 and 2000 [32]. Twenty-two of 29 tumors were nonfunctional. In 10 of 29 patients, intraoperative MRI using a 0.3-tesla vertical-field open magnet determined that the endpoint for extent of resection had been achieved after the first resection attempt, while the other 19 patients had unacceptable residual tumor on intraoperative MRI and underwent continued surgery, resulting in the achievement of the planned endpoint for extent of resection in all 29 surgeries. Operative time was extended in all cases by at least 20 min. Gross total resection was defined as removal of all tumor on MRI, recognizing that 94% of all macroadenomas demonstrate some degree of dural invasion [33], and occurred in 16 tumors overall and in 10 of the 19 tumors that underwent continued exploration after MRI. While the findings are encouraging for decreasing the incidence of residual postoperative tumor, determining whether the use of intraoperative MRI decreases long-term recurrence will require a longer follow-up in a larger group of patients.

Because of the side effects of radiotherapy for pituitary adenomas, which can include progressive pituitary failure, radiation necrosis of the optic apparatus or hypothalamus, and induction of a second CNS tumor [34–38], a British group conducted a phase I/II trial investigating systemic preoperative administration of the photosensitizing drug Photofrin followed by photodynamic therapy 48 and 24 h before surgery in the treatment of 12 patients with recurrent pituitary adenomas (8 nonfunctional, 4 secretory tumors) that had already undergone surgery and radiotherapy [39]. All 7 tumors measured at 6 months exhibited volume reduction on MRI (average 66% of preoperative volume). The only toxicity was skin sensitivity to direct sunlight early in the study in 1 patient. Although nonrandomized, the results suggest that this modality may offer some benefit to patients who have exhausted other therapeutic options.

Vestibular Schwannomas (Acoustic Neuromas)

Because of their relatively slow growth rate, the challenging nature of their microsurgical resection, and documented good outcomes with nonsurgical radiation-based approaches, the management of vestibular schwannomas (also called acoustic neuromas) is one of the more controversial topics in neurosurgery. Unfortunately, differences in short- and long-term outcomes between treatment options have only been investigated in studies producing type III or

IV evidence. A recent literature review found 111 articles reporting outcomes after acoustic neuroma management from 1977 to 2000, with 78 concerning surgery (73 type III, 5 type IV), 20 concerning radiosurgery (12 type III, 8 type IV), and 9 concerning conservative management (7 type III, 2 type IV) [40].

The first decision to be made is whether active treatment is called for, because conservative management ('watch and wait') is an appropriate course for many patients. The rationale for conservative management is that certain vestibular schwannomas may undergo a prolonged period of no growth or very slow growth, and the risks and side effects of surgery or radiation might be avoidable in this population. However, factors that identify which tumors will grow are poorly defined. A recent review of published studies attempted to identify which tumors are appropriate for conservative management [41]. The review analyzed 21 studies published between 1989 and 2003, comprising 1,345 patients followed from 0.1 to 18.0 years. The average age was 62 years, consistent with the fact that advanced age was the most common selection criterion authors advanced for conservative management. Interestingly, the studies varied significantly in the way in which tumor growth was assessed, underscoring the need for uniform criteria in studies of conservative management or active treatments for vestibular schwannomas. While nearly all studies relied on MRI, 5 studies measured only the extracanicular dimension, 7 studies measured both the intra- and extracanicular dimension, and the remainder did not specify which portion was measured. Seven studies used the single greatest tumor diameter as a measure of tumor size, while 10 studies used the average of two or more dimensions. Thirteen studies used linear measurements only, while only 3 studies attempted volumetric estimates using either three dimensions or the square of two dimensions. Because of the limited use of volumetric estimates, the authors of the review compiled linear data from the studies, finding that the initial tumor size of conservatively managed tumors was 12 mm on average, consistent with conservative management being applied to small tumors. The average growth rate was 2 mm in largest dimension per year, with a range of 0–10 mm per year. Hearing was preserved over follow-up in 49%, and lost in 51%. In 10 studies comprising 620 patients, no predictive factors could be identified for tumor growth. In 4 studies comprising 255 patients, positive growth at 1 year predicted future growth. One study of 119 patients concluded that an initial tumor size greater than 20 mm predicted earlier tumor growth. No studies succeeded in identifying predictive factors for hearing loss. Twenty percent of the patients who were initially followed later required either radiation or surgery due to growth or development of additional symptoms, the nature of which was not consistently specified. The authors compared these pooled findings to those in 64 of their own patients who were managed conservatively between 1995 and 2002. Their results were in general agreement with the literature review, including a 22% failure rate of conservative treatment. They concluded that conservative management is an acceptable option for properly selected patients, primarily older patients with smaller tumors that constituted the majority of conservatively managed patients in these studies, while acknowledging the selection bias in the group of patients for whom conservative management was recommended. However, given the lack of reliable predictive factors for growth, conservatively managed patients all warrant serial imaging and close follow-up.

Once conservative management is no longer an option, or for patients who desire active treatment immediately upon diagnosis, the next choice becomes surgery versus radiosurgery or fractionated stereotactic radiotherapy. Four studies used a retrospective cohort methodology to compare outcomes after radiosurgery to surgical resection for vestibular schwannoma patients. The first study compared 87 patients with unoperated vestibular schwannoma with a mean diameter of 3 cm or less managed with radiosurgery versus surgery during 1990–1991 at the University of Pittsburgh [42]. Patients in the surgical group were younger (51 vs. 62 years, $p < 0.001$), but tumor sizes were similar. At a median follow-up of 36 months, patients having radiosurgery were more likely to have normal facial function and preservation of useful hearing. Hospital length of stay, return to independent functioning, and treatment expense were less with radiosurgery ($p < 0.001$). Another study compared 53 surgical patients at a center in Rotterdam to 92 radiosurgery patients at an institute in Sweden between 1990 and 1995 [43]. Radiosurgery was more cost-effective, and radiosurgery patients self-reported greater levels of physical function. Another study reviewed 96 vestibular schwannoma patients having radiosurgery versus microsurgery from 1993 to 2000 at a Houston hospital [44]. Patients having surgery were younger, had larger tumors, and a longer median follow-up compared to the radiosurgery group. Radiosurgery proved more effective at hearing preservation (58 vs. 14%, $p = 0.01$). Patients undergoing microsurgery had longer hospital stays ($p < 0.01$) and more perioperative complications (48 vs. 5%, $p < 0.01$). A fourth study compared 97 patients with small- to medium-sized vestibular schwannomas having radiosurgery from 1992 to 1998 with 110 vestibular schwannoma patients having surgery from 1983 to 1990 at a French hospital [45]. Once again, radiosurgery patients were older. New facial weakness was more common in the surgical group (37 vs. 0%). Hearing preservation was more common in the radiosurgery group (70 vs. 38%). These four studies provide consistent level 3 evidence showing that, in the short term, radiosurgery provides better outcomes than surgical resection for patients with small- to medium-sized vestibular schwannomas that have not undergone previous surgery.

Theoretically, fractionation of the radiotherapy dose should reduce damage to late-responding neural tissues such as cranial nerves, brainstem, and cerebellum. A comparison of fractionated to single fraction radiotherapy was attempted by a German group, who compared results in treating vestibular schwannomas with stereotactic LINAC-based convergent beam radiosurgery versus fractionated stereotactic conformation beam radiotherapy [46]. All 21 treated patients experienced no further tumor growth. Four of 9 single dose-treated patients developed side effects (temporary trigeminal and facial paresthesia, hearing deterioration, and edema), while patients receiving fractionated radiation showed no side effects. Later, a Canadian group retrospectively studied vestibular schwannoma patients at a single institution treated with single-fraction stereotactic radiosurgery (45 patients receiving a single dose of 12 Gy usually prescribed to the 80% isodose line) or fractionated stereotactic radiotherapy (27 patients receiving 45 Gy in 25 fractions during 5 weeks prescribed to the 90% isodose line). The two groups were comparable in duration of median follow-up (26–27 months), age, and tumor size [47]. Both groups had 100% tumor control rate at the end of follow-up. Hearing preservation was not compared. While the single-fraction group had a 95.6% facial nerve preservation rate and the fractionated group had 100% facial preservation at the end of follow-up, the difference was not significant, indicating that a larger series of patients would need to be compared in order to determine if fractionated radiation was more effective at cranial nerve preservation.

When a decision is made to surgically treat a vestibular schwannoma, the surgical approach becomes the next decision to be made. For patients with minimal preoperative hearing (usually associated with larger tumors), the translabyrinthine approach can be considered, offering a more anterior corridor of access than the retrosigmoid approach, resulting in minimal cerebellar retraction. One study retrospectively compared outcomes in 17 patients operated on through a retrosigmoid approach to 81 patients operated on through the translabyrinthine route [48]. Mean ages and tumor sizes did not vary between the groups. One year after tumor removal via the retrosigmoid approach, 10 of 17 patients (59%) had good (House-Brackmann grade I–II) facial function and 2 (12%) had poor (grade V–VI) function. In the translabyrinthine group, 54 (68%) of 79 patients (2 patients had subtotal total tumor removal) had good facial nerve function at the end of the 1-year follow-up, and 13 (17%) continued to have poor facial function. The difference between these groups was not statistically significant ($p > 0.05$). Hearing was preserved in 4 (24%) of the 17 patients in the retrosigmoid group, and none in the translabyrinthine group.

For patients in whom hearing preservation is desired, the choice is between the middle fossa or retrosigmoid approach. A synthetic review performed in 2004 first compiled a case study of patient data entered into a prospectively designed database at the Seattle Ear Clinic, then combining this data with similar data from 11 other institutions to compare the two approaches [49]. The review focused on studies in which a percentage of tumor removal was reported and patients with partial removals were excluded. Median facial nerve results for all institutions were significantly better with the retrosigmoid approach (grade I facial nerve function rates were 95% for retrosigmoid, 81% for middle fossa), with a significant difference (Wilcoxon rank sum test, $p = 0.014$). Median hearing results trended towards better outcome with the middle fossa approach (preoperative hearing class maintained in 48% of middle fossa cases, 39% of retrosigmoid cases), but the difference was not significant (Wilcoxon rank sum test, $p > 0.5$), due in part to the fact that the reporting institution had an equal or greater effect on outcome than the choice of surgical approach.

Despite progress in functional outcome after surgical resection and a reduced incidence of major complications such as brainstem injury, cerebrospinal fluid (CSF) leaks with their associated risk of meningitis remain an important complication in the surgical management of vestibular schwannomas. A synthetic review of studies published between 1985 and 2004 found that CSF leak occurred in 10.6% of 2,273 retrosigmoid surgeries, 9.5% of 3,118 translabyrinthine surgeries, and 10.6% of 573 middle fossa surgeries, indicating that the surgical approach did not influence the risk of CSF leak [50]. Meningitis was significantly associated with CSF leak ($p < 0.05$). Age and tumor size were not associated with CSF leak.

While the goal of vestibular schwannoma surgery is tumor removal while preserving cranial nerve function, the goal of radiation treatments for vestibular schwannoma is tumor control. As a result, potential radiosurgery failures include younger patients whose tumors recur at an older age, a concern because long-term tumor control with radiosurgery remains to be investigated, and patients of any age in whom short-term control fails to be achieved. The challenges of surgery in the latter group were investigated in a case-control series comparing surgery of 9 patients with vestibular schwannomas that grew or caused new symptoms after radiotherapy to surgery of 9 nonirradiated control subjects matched for age, sex, tumor size (2.6 cm in irradiated tumors, 2.8 cm in nonirradiated tumors), and surgical approach [51]. The same surgeon performed all operations in this series. Acknowledging the bias inherent in the fact that the surgeon was always aware of which tumors were irradiated, the authors reported that surgical removal was found to be significantly more difficult in radiated vestibular schwannomas due to fibrosis and adhesion to adjacent nervous structures, particularly at the porus acusticus. Excessive scarring hindered identification of the facial nerve and added uncertainty as to the completeness of tumor removal. While gross total resection based on the surgeon's operative characterization was achieved in all nonirradiated tumors, in five of eight irradiated tumors, the final stages of dissection led to a point where scar and tumor could not be distinguished from one another, leading to uncertainty about the extent of tumor removal. Operative time was 501 min in the irradiated group compared to 407 min in the nonirradiated group ($p = 0.04$). While preoperative facial nerve function was slightly worse in the irradiated group, House-Brackmann grade 2 versus 1, the difference was not significant ($p = 0.25$). Postoperative facial nerve function was, however, significantly worse in the irradiated group, grade 4 versus 2 ($p = 0.05$), although the effect of the differing preoperative scores was not subtracted out. The authors conclude that, while poorer outcomes occur with surgical resection of irradiated vestibular schwannomas, surgical salvage of acoustic neuromas after failed radiation therapy is feasible.

In a retrospective analysis of 70 patients with acoustic neuromas, brainstem auditory evoked potentials showed gradual reversible loss [52]. Two thirds of these patients eventually suffered from anacusis as a result of tumor removal [52]. Based on the hypothesis that disturbed microcirculation secondary to nerve edema and vasospasm of the vasa nervorum causes hearing loss in these patients, a German group initiated a prospective randomized trial of vasoactive medications in the postoperative period after surgical removal of acoustic neuromas [53]. In all 41 patients, the cochlear nerve was preserved during surgery. Twenty patients received no postoperative medication other than dexamethasone, while 21 patients received a nimodipine-soaked gelfoam pad during surgery, followed by intravenous calcium channel blocker nimodipine immediately after the surgical procedure and a 6% solution of intravenous hydroxyethyl starch (HES) 24 h after surgery. Nimodipine and HES were given for an average of 9 days. Both groups were comparable in age, tumor size, and preoperative hearing. In the steroid-only group, 70% had documented postoperative anacusis (30% immediate, 40% delayed) 3 months after surgery, exceeding the 33.3% incidence of postoperative anacusis (23.8% immediate, 9.5% delayed) in patients receiving HES and nimodipine, with a significant difference ($p < 0.05$). No significant side effects were reported. The authors recommend using vasoactive mediations to improve hearing outcome following neurosurgical removal of vestibular schwannomas.

Like the other benign adult brain tumors described above, double-blind studies to evaluate therapies for acoustic neuroma have not yet been undertaken, but could contribute much to their management. Although radiotherapy alone is inappropriate treatment in most circumstances for larger tumors (>3 cm), which currently require surgical decompression, there are decisions to be made in the management of smaller vestibular schwannomas in which either option could be ethically undertaken in a clinical trial. For example, smaller tumors (<1 cm) at diagnosis could ethically be randomized prospectively into no treatment or radiosurgery arms. It would also be ethical to randomize tumors of intermediate size with evidence of radiographic growth into radiosurgery or surgery groups. However, a randomized study would still be difficult to perform because of patient preferences and difficult to interpret because the experience of each individual surgical team influences outcome.

Neurofibromatosis Type 2

Patients with neurofibromatosis type 2 (NF2) develop benign brain tumors throughout life, including bilateral vestibular schwannomas, typically seen at presentation, in addition to other intracranial tumors such as schwannomas and meningiomas. The management of vestibular schwannomas in these patients is particularly challenging. Not only are they at risk for complete deafness and other associated functional disabilities caused by bilateral tumors such as facial weakness, but many NF2 patients harbor other intracranial neoplasms that may further complicate management. Additional challenges arise from the findings that vestibular schwannomas in NF2 patients have a shorter doubling time (29.2 months) than sporadic vestibular schwannomas (35.2 months) [54]; left- and right-sided vestibular schwannomas in NF2 patients with bilateral vestibular schwannomas grow at similar rates [55]; and vestibular schwannomas in NF2 patients tend to invade rather than displace the cochlear nerve [56]. These findings make conservative management of vestibular schwannomas in NF2 patients particularly challenging, although a large case series attempting to identify factors that predict tumor growth during conservative management is lacking in NF2 vestibular schwannomas.

Given the particular importance of hearing preservation in this population with bilateral risks and given the benefit of radiosurgery in short-term hearing preservation described above, radiation has been investigated in the management of vestibular schwannomas associated with NF2. This was done through a pair of case series studies providing level 4 evidence. The first study retrospectively reviewed the experience at the University of Pittsburgh between 1987 and 1997 in treating 40 NF2 patients with 45 vestibular schwannomas treated with stereotactically guided radiosurgery using the gamma knife [56]. Thirteen patients had undergone a median of two prior resections. The mean tumor volume at radiosurgery was 4.8 ml, and the mean tumor margin dose was 15 Gy (range 12–20 Gy). The overall tumor control rate was 98%. During a median follow-up of 36 months, 16 tumors (36%) regressed, 28 (62%) remained unchanged, and 1 (2%) grew. Three patients underwent surgical resection after radiosurgery. Useful hearing was preserved in 43% of patients, and normal facial nerve function was preserved in 81% of patients. The authors conclude that, while many NF2 vestibular schwannomas become large enough to require surgical decompression, radiosurgery offers effective control with moderate hearing preservation compared to surgery and good preservation of facial function for smaller vestibular schwannomas or for larger ones that have undergone subtotal resection. Another study 1 year later retrospectively analyzed 20 NF2 patients with bilateral vestibular schwannomas treated unilaterally with stereotactic gamma knife radiosurgery at a center in Japan [57]. The tumor regression rate was 60% at 36 months. Tumors contralateral to the treated tumor were enlarged in 40% of patients. Hearing preservation occurred in one third of patients. Facial nerve deterioration occurred in 10%. The authors conclude that, given the similar growth rates of bilateral tumors in NF2 patients, the contralateral tumors in these unilaterally treated patients offer internal controls validating the benefits of radiosurgery in NF2 patients. Although hearing preservation was difficult, facial nerve preservation was common.

Improved neurofunctional outcome may occur if fractionated stereotactic radiosurgery is used to treat vestibular schwannomas in NF2 patients. One study of fractionated stereotactic radiosurgery in vestibular schwannoma treatment at a single German institution included 41 patients with sporadic vestibular schwannomas and 10 NF2 patients with bilateral tumors [58]. All NF2 patients had undergone treatment of the contralateral side (9 with surgery, 1 with radiosurgery) with subsequent hearing loss and facial nerve weakness. Mean tumor volume in NF2 patients was $16.0\,cm^3$, almost twice that of non-NF2 tumors. One of 10 NF2 patients experienced moderate worsening of facial dysfunction. Hearing preservation in NF2 patients was 56% at 2 and 5 years, compared to 100% at 2 and 5 years in non-NF2 vestibular schwannomas ($p = 0.0002$). Although lacking matched controls, the authors conclude that fractionated stereotactic radiosurgery offers good short-term control of vestibular schwannomas in NF2, with less risk to hearing and facial function than surgery or radiosurgery.

Conclusions

While anatomically, histologically, and clinically distinct, benign adult brain tumors share the fact that evidence from randomized trials is mostly lacking. This is a challenge that affects all of neuro-oncology, particularly those nonaggressive tumors which must be followed for a decade or more before an appropriate endpoint can be reached. Using the existing evidence, which is level 3 or below, a better understanding of the advantages of different treatment options can be obtained.

References

1 CBTRUS: Statistical Report: Primary Brain Tumors in the United States, 1997–2001. Hinsdale, Central Brain Tumor Registry of the United States, 2004.
2 Monson JP: The epidemiology of endocrine tumours. Endocr Relat Cancer 2000;7:29–36.

3 Wara WM, Sheline GE, Newman H, Townsend JJ, Boldrey EB: Radiation therapy of meningiomas. Am J Roentgenol Radium Ther Nucl Med 1975;123:453–458.
4 Harner SG, Laws ER Jr: Clinical findings in patients with acoustic neurinoma. Mayo Clin Proc 1983;58:721–728.
5 Drummond KJ, Zhu JJ, Black PM: Meningiomas: updating basic science, management, and outcome. Neurologist 2004;10:113–130.
6 Kuratsu J, Kochi M, Ushio Y: Incidence and clinical features of asymptomatic meningiomas. J Neurosurg 2000;92:766–770.
7 Simpson D: The recurrence of intracranial meningiomas after surgical treatment. J Neurochem 1957;20:22–39.
8 Condra KS, Buatti JM, Mendenhall WM, Friedman WA, Marcus RB Jr, Rhoton AL: Benign meningiomas: primary treatment selection affects survival. Int J Radiat Oncol Biol Phys 1997;39: 427–436.
9 Mathiesen T, Lindquist C, Kihlstrom L, Karlsson B: Recurrence of cranial base meningiomas. Neurosurgery 1996;39:2–9.
10 Borovich B, Doron Y, Braun J, Guilburd JN, Zaaroor M, Goldsher D, et al: Recurrence of intracranial meningiomas: the role played by regional multicentricity. 2. Clinical and radiological aspects. J Neurosurg 1986;65:168–171.
11 Borovich B, Doron Y: Recurrence of intracranial meningiomas: the role played by regional multicentricity. J Neurosurg 1986;64:58–63.
12 Kinjo T, al-Mefty O, Kanaan I: Grade zero removal of supratentorial convexity meningiomas. Neurosurgery 1993;33:394–399.
13 Rohringer M, Sutherland GR, Louw DF, Sima AA: Incidence and clinicopathological features of meningioma. J Neurosurg 1989;71:665–672.
14 Black P, Kathiresan S, Chung W: Meningioma surgery in the elderly: a case-control study assessing morbidity and mortality. Acta Neurochir (Wien) 1998;140:1013–1017.
15 Pollock BE, Stafford SL, Utter A, Giannini C, Schreiner SA: Stereotactic radiosurgery provides equivalent tumor control to Simpson Grade 1 resection for patients with small- to medium-size meningiomas. Int J Radiat Oncol Biol Phys 2003;55:1000–1005.
16 Grunberg SM RC, Townsend J, Ahmadi J, Feun L, Fredericks R, Russell C, Kabbinavar F, Barger GR, Stelzer KJ: Phase III double-blind randomized placebo-controlled study of mifepristone (RU) for the treatment of unresectable meningioma (abstract 222). American Society of Clinical Oncology (ASCO) 37th Annual Meeting, San Francisco, 2001, p 56a.
17 Muhr C, Gudjonsson O, Lilja A, Hartman M, Zhang ZJ, Langstrom B: Meningioma treated with interferon-alpha, evaluated with [(11)C]-*L*-methionine positron emission tomography. Clin Cancer Res 2001;7:2269–2276.
18 Chamberlain MC, Tsao-Wei DD, Groshen S: Temozolomide for treatment-resistant recurrent meningioma. Neurology 2004;62:1210–1212.
19 Swinnen L, Barger G: Phase II study of hydroxyurea in patients with unresectable benign meningioma. Protocol ID SWOG-S9811, 2005; www.clinicaltrials.gov
20 Schloffer H: Erfolgreiche Operation eines Hypophysentumors auf nasalem Wege. Wien Klin Wochenschr 1907;20:621–624.
21 Molitch ME, Elton RL, Blackwell RE, Caldwell B, Chang RJ, Jaffe R, et al: Bromocriptine as primary therapy for prolactin-secreting macroadenomas: results of a prospective multicenter study. J Clin Endocrinol Metab 1985;60:698–705.
22 Passos VQ, Souza JJ, Musolino NR, Bronstein MD: Long-term follow-up of prolactinomas: normoprolactinemia after bromocriptine withdrawal. J Clin Endocrinol Metab 2002;87:3578–3582.
23 Colao A, Lombardi G: Growth-hormone and prolactin excess. Lancet 1998;352:1455–1461.
24 Molitch ME: Medical management of prolactin-secreting pituitary adenomas. Pituitary 2002;5: 55–65.
25 Katznelson L, Alexander JM, Klibanski A: Clinical review 45: clinically nonfunctioning pituitary adenomas. J Clin Endocrinol Metab 1993;76:1089–1094.
26 Shihadeh ED, Ryu S, Bogart JA, Chung CT, Rogers M: Outcome of radiation therapy alone and post-operative radiation for non-functioning pituitary adenoma (abstract 589). American Society of Clinical Oncology (ASCO) 35th Annual Meeting, Atlanta, 1999, p 153a.

27 Woollons AC, Hunn MK, Rajapakse YR, Toomath R, Hamilton DA, Conaglen JV, et al: Nonfunctioning pituitary adenomas: indications for postoperative radiotherapy. Clin Endocrinol (Oxf) 2000;53:713–717.
28 Losa M, Franzin A, Mangili F, Terreni MR, Barzaghi R, Veglia F, et al: Proliferation index of nonfunctioning pituitary adenomas: correlations with clinical characteristics and long-term follow-up results. Neurosurgery 2000;47:1313–1319.
29 Picozzi P, Losa M, Mortini P, Valle MA, Franzin A, Attuati L, et al: Radiosurgery and the prevention of regrowth of incompletely removed nonfunctioning pituitary adenomas. J Neurosurg 2005;102(suppl):71–74.
30 Swearingen B, Barker FG 2nd, Katznelson L, Biller BM, Grinspoon S, Klibanski A, et al: Longterm mortality after transsphenoidal surgery and adjunctive therapy for acromegaly. J Clin Endocrinol Metab 1998;83:3419–3426.
31 Landolt AM, Haller D, Lomax N, Scheib S, Schubiger O, Siegfried J, et al: Stereotactic radiosurgery for recurrent surgically treated acromegaly: comparison with fractionated radiotherapy. J Neurosurg 1998;88:1002–1008.
32 Bohinski RJ, Warnick RE, Gaskill-Shipley MF, Zuccarello M, van Loveren HR, Kormos DW, et al: Intraoperative magnetic resonance imaging to determine the extent of resection of pituitary macroadenomas during transsphenoidal microsurgery. Neurosurgery 2001;49:1133–1144.
33 Selman WR, Laws ER Jr, Scheithauer BW, Carpenter SM: The occurrence of dural invasion in pituitary adenomas. J Neurosurg 1986;64:402–407.
34 al-Mefty O, Kersh JE, Routh A, Smith RR: The long-term side effects of radiation therapy for benign brain tumors in adults. J Neurosurg 1990;73:502–512.
35 Bieri S, Sklar C, Constine L, Bernier J: Late effects of radiotherapy on the neuroendocrine system. Cancer Radiother 1997;1:706–716.
36 Guy J, Mancuso A, Beck R, Moster ML, Sedwick LA, Quisling RG, et al: Radiation-induced optic neuropathy: a magnetic resonance imaging study. J Neurosurg 1991;74:426–432.
37 Plataniotis GA, Kouvaris JR, Vlahos L, Papavasiliou C: Radiation therapy alone for growth hormone-producing pituitary adenomas. Acta Oncol 1998;37:97–99.
38 Lillehei KO, Kirschman DL, Kleinschmidt-DeMasters BK, Ridgway EC: Reassessment of the role of radiation therapy in the treatment of endocrine-inactive pituitary macroadenomas. Neurosurgery 1998;43:432–439.
39 Marks PV, Belchetz PE, Saxena A, Igbaseimokumo U, Thomson S, Nelson M, et al: Effect of photodynamic therapy on recurrent pituitary adenomas: clinical phase I/II trial – an early report. Br J Neurosurg 2000;14:317–325.
40 Nikolopoulos TP, O'Donoghue GM: Acoustic neuroma management: an evidence-based medicine approach. Otol Neurotol 2002;23:534–541.
41 Smouha EE, Yoo M, Mohr K, Davis RP: Conservative management of acoustic neuroma: a metaanalysis and proposed treatment algorithm. Laryngoscope 2005;115:450–454.
42 Pollock BE, Lunsford LD, Kondziolka D, Flickinger JC, Bissonette DJ, Kelsey SF, et al: Outcome analysis of acoustic neuroma management: a comparison of microsurgery and stereotactic radiosurgery. Neurosurgery 1995;36:215–229.
43 van Roijen L, Nijs HG, Avezaat CJ, Karlsson G, Linquist C, Pauw KH, et al: Costs and effects of microsurgery versus radiosurgery in treating acoustic neuroma. Acta Neurochir (Wien) 1997;139: 942–948.
44 Karpinos M, Teh BS, Zeck O, Carpenter LS, Phan C, Mai WY, et al: Treatment of acoustic neuroma: stereotactic radiosurgery vs. microsurgery. Int J Radiat Oncol Biol Phys 2002;54:1410–1421.
45 Regis J, Pellet W, Delsanti C, Dufour H, Roche PH, Thomassin JM, et al: Functional outcome after gamma knife surgery or microsurgery for vestibular schwannomas. J Neurosurg 2002;97: 1091–1100.
46 Becker G, Schlegel W, Major J, Grote EH, Bamberg M: Stereotactic convergent beam radiosurgery versus stereotactic conformation beam radiotherapy. Acta Neurochir Suppl 1995;63:44–51.
47 Chung HT, Ma R, Toyota B, Clark B, Robar J, McKenzie M: Audiologic and treatment outcomes after linear accelerator-based stereotactic irradiation for acoustic neuroma. Int J Radiat Oncol Biol Phys 2004;59:1116–1121.

48 Mamikoglu B, Esquivel CR, Wiet RJ: Comparison of facial nerve function results after translabyrinthine and retrosigmoid approach in medium-sized tumors. Arch Otolaryngol Head Neck Surg 2003;129:429–431.
49 Mangham CA Jr: Retrosigmoid versus middle fossa surgery for small vestibular schwannomas. Laryngoscope 2004;114:1455–1461.
50 Selesnick SH, Liu JC, Jen A, Newman J: The incidence of cerebrospinal fluid leak after vestibular schwannoma surgery. Otol Neurotol 2004;25:387–393.
51 Limb CJ, Long DM, Niparko JK: Acoustic neuromas after failed radiation therapy: challenges of surgical salvage. Laryngoscope 2005;115:93–98.
52 Neu M, Strauss C, Romstock J, Bischoff B, Fahlbusch R: The prognostic value of intraoperative BAEP patterns in acoustic neurinoma surgery. Clin Neurophysiol 1999;110:1935–1941.
53 Strauss C, Bischoff B, Neu M, Berg M, Fahlbusch R, Romstock J: Vasoactive treatment for hearing preservation in acoustic neuroma surgery. J Neurosurg 2001;95:771–777.
54 Ogawa K, Kanzaki J, Ogawa S, Yamamoto M, Ikeda S, Shiobara R: The growth rate of acoustic neuromas. Acta Otolaryngol Suppl 1991;487:157–163.
55 Mautner VF, Baser ME, Thakkar SD, Feigen UM, Friedman JM, Kluwe L: Vestibular schwannoma growth in patients with neurofibromatosis type 2: a longitudinal study. J Neurosurg 2002;96: 223–228.
56 Subach BR, Kondziolka D, Lunsford LD, Bissonette DJ, Flickinger JC, Maitz AH: Stereotactic radiosurgery in the management of acoustic neuromas associated with neurofibromatosis type 2. J Neurosurg 1999;90:815–822.
57 Kida Y, Kobayashi T, Tanaka T, Mori Y: Radiosurgery for bilateral neurinomas associated with neurofibromatosis type 2. Surg Neurol 2000;53:383–390.
58 Fuss M, Debus J, Lohr F, Huber P, Rhein B, Engenhart-Cabillic R, et al: Conventionally fractionated stereotactic radiotherapy (FSRT) for acoustic neuromas. Int J Radiat Oncol Biol Phys 2000;48:1381–1387.

Manish Aghi, MD
Neurosurgical Service
Massachusetts General Hospital
White Building, Room 502, 55 Fruit Street
Boston, MA 02114 (USA)
Tel. +1 617 726 2241, Fax +1 617 726 4814, E-Mail maghi@partners.org

Pollock BE (ed): Guiding Neurosurgery by Evidence.
Prog Neurol Surg. Basel, Karger, 2006, vol 19, pp 97–106

Pediatric Neurosurgery

Cormac O. Maher[a], *Aaron A. Cohen-Gadol*[b], *Corey Raffel*[b]

[a]Department of Neurosurgery, Children's Hospital Boston, Boston, Mass.,
[b]Department of Neurosurgery, Mayo Clinic, Rochester, Minn., USA

Abstract

Randomized controlled trials of neurosurgical procedures involving children have been organized infrequently; as a consequence, the majority of pediatric neurosurgical practice is not supported by class I data. Furthermore, many trials that have been reported suffer from serious methodological shortcomings such as insufficient power and poor statistical analysis. Finally, several trials of neurosurgical techniques that are frequently performed on children have either excluded children from participation or include an insufficient number of children to draw strong conclusions. Despite these shortcomings, pediatric neurosurgery, like all fields in medicine, is gradually moving towards a more stringent evidence-based medicine standard. This chapter will attempt to summarize the recent progress that has been made in this area.

Hydrocephalus

Hydrocephalus is the most common disease that is treated by pediatric neurosurgeons. As such, it has also been the subject of the largest number of clinical trials (table 1). Two recent trials of ventriculoperitoneal shunt placement have evaluated the role of valve type and endoscopic-assisted placement of ventricular catheters. The Pediatric Shunt Design trial compared a large number of patients that were randomized according to valve type [1]. This trial demonstrated a lack of difference between three commonly available and utilized valve models. The Endoscopic Shunt Insertion trial compared a large group of patients that were randomized to ventriculoperitoneal shunt placement either with or without endoscopic assistance during proximal catheter positioning [2]. These authors found that endoscopic shunt placement did not decrease the incidence of shunt failure compared with the standard technique.

Table 1. Pediatric hydrocephalus trials

Authors	Year	Randomization	n	Conclusion(s)
Drake et al. [1]	1998	differential pressure valve Delta valve (PS Medical) Orbis-Sigma valve (NMT Cordis)	114 115 115	no difference in incidence of shunt failure
Zentner et al. [16b]	1995	perioperative antibiotics no perioperative antibiotics	67 62	perioperative antibiotics associated with lower infection rate (not statistically significant)
Kestle et al. [2]	2003	endoscopic VPS insertion standard VPS insertion	194 199	endoscope-assisted shunt placement did not decrease the incidence of shunt failure
Govender et al. [17]	2003	antibiotic impregnated shunt control shunt	50 60	the antibiotic impregnated shunt was protective against early staphylococcal shunt infections
Haines and Taylor [9]	1982	perioperative antibiotics no perioperative antibiotics	35 39	perioperative antibiotics associated with lower infection rate (not statistically significant)
Bayston [4]	1975	perioperative antibiotics no perioperative antibiotics	54 78	perioperative antibiotics associated with lower infection rate (not statistically significant)
Yogev et al. [15]	1983	perioperative antibiotics no perioperative antibiotics	106 84	perioperative antibiotics associated with lower infection rate (not statistically significant)
Lambert et al. [10]	1984	perioperative antibiotics no perioperative antibiotics	24 44	perioperative antibiotics associated with lower infection rate (not statistically significant)
Odio et al. [11]	1984	perioperative antibiotics no perioperative antibiotics	18 17	perioperative antibiotics associated with lower infection rate (not statistically significant)
Wang et al. [14]	1984	perioperative antibiotics no perioperative antibiotics	55 65	perioperative antibiotics associated with lower infection rate (not statistically significant)
Blomstedt [5]	1985	perioperative antibiotics no perioperative antibiotics	62 60	perioperative antibiotics associated with statistically significant lower infection rate
Schmidt et al. [13]	1985	perioperative antibiotics no perioperative antibiotics	79 73	perioperative antibiotics associated with higher infection rate (not statistically significant)

Table 1. (continued)

Authors	Year	Randomization	n	Conclusion(s)
Djindjian et al. [7]	1986	perioperative antibiotics no perioperative antibiotics	30 30	perioperative antibiotics associated with lower infection rate (not statistically significant)
Reider et al. [12]	1987	perioperative antibiotics no perioperative antibiotics	31 32	perioperative antibiotics associated with lower infection rate (not statistically significant)
Blum et al. [6]	1989	perioperative antibiotics no perioperative antibiotics	50 50	perioperative antibiotics associated with lower infection rate (not statistically significant)
Walters et al. [16]	1992	perioperative antibiotics no perioperative antibiotics	130 113	perioperative antibiotics associated with lower infection rate (not statistically significant)

VPS = Ventriculoperitoneal shunt.

Many studies have evaluated the utility of perioperative antimicrobial prophylaxis for shunt placement. In a review of the literature, Langley et al. [3] identified 12 published trials, including an aggregate of 1,359 patients, with random allocation to antibiotic prophylaxis versus no antibiotic prophylaxis for shunt surgery [4–16]. Most of these trials enrolled children only or all age groups. Langley et al. found that, when examined individually, only 1 of the 12 published trials found that antibiotics reduced the risk of shunt infection to a statistically significant degree and one trial [13] actually reported a higher infection rate in the antibiotic-treated group. A meta-analysis of these 12 trials, however, found that antibiotic use led to a very significant decrease in the risk of infection. This demonstrates the value of meta-analysis in the neurosurgical literature. We may suppose that most of the studies failed to show 'significance' when evaluated individually because of insufficient power arising from small sample sizes, a problem that is endemic in neurosurgical trials.

The use of antibiotic-impregnated shunts in an attempt to decrease the rate of shunt infections is relatively new and has been the subject of only one controlled trial to date [17]. This study suggests that the use of antibiotic-impregnated shunts reduces the incidence of early staphylococcal shunt infections.

Much of the data on the management of external ventricular drains are derived from trials that are mostly or entirely composed of adult patients [18, 19]. Consequently, the application of these data to the pediatric population is a matter of debate.

Table 2. Epilepsy surgery trials

Authors	Year	Randomization	n	Conclusion(s)
Wyler et al. [22]	1995[a]	partial hippocampectomy	34	total hippocampectomy associated with significantly superior seizure
		total hippocampectomy	36	outcome (69 vs. 38% seizure-free) without increased neuropsychological morbidity
Salinsky et al. [26]	1995	high-level stimulation (VNS)	54	high-level VNS associated with significantly decreased seizure
		low-level stimulation (VNS)	60	frequency compared with low stimulation (24.5 vs. 6.1% reduction)
Handforth et al. [27]	1998	high-level stimulation (VNS)	94	high-level VNS associated with significantly decreased seizure
		low-level stimulation (VNS)	102	frequency compared with low stimulation (28 vs. 15% reduction)
Wiebe et al.[b] [20]	2001	temporal lobectomy	40	significantly greater seizure freedom in surgical group (58%) versus
		medical treatment alone	40	medical group (8%); at 1 year quality of life also greater in surgical group

VNS = Vagus nerve stimulation.
[a]No pediatric patients.
[b]All patients >16 years old.

Pediatric Epilepsy

Although temporal lobectomy has been an established treatment option for temporal lobe epilepsy for many years, the first randomized controlled trial of surgery for temporal lobe epilepsy was not reported until 2001 (table 2) [20]. In this trial Wiebe et al. assigned 40 patients to immediate surgery and 40 patients to medical treatment for 1 year (which was the expected waiting time for surgery at their institution). As expected, the surgical group enjoyed a greater probability of freedom from seizures as well as improvements in quality of life. These data have led to new practice parameters from the American Academy of Neurology [21]. Although all patients in this trial were greater than 16 years of age, there are no data to indicate that pediatric patients should be treated differently. Therefore, this study remains the best available examination of a common intervention in pediatric neurosurgical practice.

The extent of medial temporal resection in anterior temporal lobectomy procedures has also been the subject of a randomized trial [22]. Wyler et al. [22]

randomized 70 patients, all undergoing anterior temporal lobectomy for seizures, according to the length of hippocampal removal. This group found that resection of hippocampus to the level of the tectal plate ('total hippocampectomy') resulted in a better seizure outcome compared with removal of the hippocampus to the level of the cerebral peduncle ('partial hippocampectomy'). Although no children were included in this trial, its conclusions are likely to extend to the pediatric population.

The First International Vagus Nerve Stimulation Study Group demonstrated the effectiveness of vagal nerve stimulation in the treatment of partial seizures [23–26]. In this well-designed study, patients were randomized to receive either high-level or low-level vagus nerve stimulation. In this way, these authors were able to bypass the difficulties that are associated with randomizing for surgery versus no surgery. In the second randomized-controlled trial of vagus nerve stimulation for refractory epilepsy, Handforth et al. [27] also compared high-level to low-level stimulation and found a benefit with the former. Despite the frequent application of this treatment to children with refractory epilepsy, pediatric patients comprised only a minority of patients enrolled in these trials.

Pediatric Brain Tumors

Most of the trials concern the utility of chemotherapy or radiation therapy and do not randomize according to surgical procedure. Nevertheless, most contemporary trials evaluating the effectiveness of adjunctive therapies do make a surgical procedure (biopsy, partial resection, subtotal resection or gross total resection) a mandatory condition of enrollment.

Several trials that were focused on randomizing patients according to adjunctive postoperative treatments have enrolled patients regardless of the extent of surgical resection. Although surgical treatment was not randomized or controlled in these studies, they informed current care guidelines for the surgical treatment of pediatric brain tumors. For example, in a randomized controlled trial examining postoperative chemotherapy without irradiation following surgical resection of ependymoma, Grill et al. [28] found a significant difference in outcomes between subtotal and gross totally resected ependymomas. Similarly, Wolff et al. [29] have reported on a randomized controlled trial evaluating the role of specific chemotherapy regimens in children with grade 3 or 4 gliomas. Although surgery was not randomized, these authors found that the extent of surgical resection was the most important prognostic factor.

Wisoff et al. [30, 31] performed a post hoc analysis of the Children's Cancer Group trial number CCG-945 which was conceived in order to compare the efficacy of two different chemotherapy regimens. These authors found that, among patients enrolled in this trial, those undergoing more extensive resections exhibited longer survival times and progression-free survivals. Although this study was based on a prospectively accrued patient population, it is subject to a variety of biases due to the retrospective analysis [32]. For instance, the determination of the extent of resection as well as the definition of groups for comparison are both subject to bias. In addition, the extent of surgery is not randomized in any of these studies, therefore even stringent statistical analysis may not eliminate important confounding variables.

Spasticity

The two most utilized neurosurgical treatments for spasticity, baclofen pumps and dorsal rhizotomy, have both been the subject of randomized trials. Armstrong et al. [33] have reported on a series of patients with baclofen pumps in which all study patients were selected as a result of a trial of intrathecal baclofen injections compared with intrathecal saline injections. Although the study patients were selected for pump implantation based on positive results of this double-blind trial, the utility of baclofen pump placement was reported as a case series without a control group. Other trials of baclofen pumps have primarily studied adults [34, 35].

The utility of selective dorsal rhizotomy has been the subject of three randomized controlled trials [36–38]. Although sample sizes were small, each of these trials were well-organized and suggested a potential beneficial effect for this operation. The report of McLaughlin et al. [36], the largest of the three studies, suggested that the decrease in spasticity in the surgical arm of the trial was not functionally important. The differing results may be a result of variations in physical therapy regimens between the studies. Further clarification may be added by either a larger trial or meta-analysis [39].

Fetal Surgery

Since the publication of initial results from the International Fetal Surgery Registry, a nonrandomized prospective clinical database of fetal surgery procedures, in utero surgery for the correction of hydrocephalus and myelomeningocele has remained controversial [40]. Farmer et al. [41] have reported on a case control study evaluating different methods of in utero myelomeningocele repair, preferring ‘open’ techniques to fetoscopic methods. This study, however, did not address the central question in fetal surgery: does in utero repair have any additional benefit compared with postnatal repair? The first trial that was organized to address this question failed for methodological reasons [42, 43]. Currently, patients are being accrued for the Management of Myelomeningocele Study (MOMS). MOMS is a prospective, randomized trial for in utero surgical repair of myelomeningocele [44]. Fetuses enrolled in this ongoing trial are randomly assigned to either in utero repair of the myelomeningocele at between 19 and 25 weeks' gestation or cesarean delivery followed by standard surgical treatment [44]. The primary endpoints of this trial are the need for a shunt procedure at 1 year and mortality. Results are expected in approximately 2006 [44].

Pediatric Head Injuries

Pediatric head injury management has been the subject of two recent trials. In a prospective randomized trial of 102 children following moderate to severe head injury, Young et al. [45] showed that prophylactic treatment with phenytoin did not reduce the rate of early (within 48 h) posttraumatic seizures. The patients in this trial were not selected or stratified according to established risks for posttraumatic seizures such as the presence of a large contusion, therefore the conclusions may not apply to patients that are thought to be at increased risk.

In an attempt to evaluate the role of decompressive craniectomy in children with elevated intracranial pressure following head injury, Taylor et al. [46] randomized children with elevated intracranial pressure following trauma to either craniectomy or medical management alone. Although the craniectomy did appear to be beneficial, the small number of patients (27) that were randomized limits the information that may be derived from this trial.

Conclusions

Clearly, the vast majority of current pediatric neurosurgical practice is not supported by evidence-based medicine standards. Rather, practice patterns have been established that are based mostly on the uncontrolled reported experiences with consecutive patient series. These reports are, for the most part, uncontrolled and analyzed retrospectively.

This reliance on class III evidence within the field of pediatric neurosurgery does appear to be slowly shifting in favor of an increased willingness to organize and participate in randomized clinical trials. In the area of pediatric brain tumor treatments, our progress towards proper trial methodology has been accelerated by the involvement of multicenter and multispecialty clinical consortia such as and the Children's Oncology Group [COG; a merger of the

Pediatric Oncology Group (POG) and the Children's Cancer Study Group]. The evidence in favor of antibiotic prophylaxis during shunting procedures is similarly robust. Although the publication of the shunt design trial results represents an important step, many other important questions regarding the management of hydrocephalus remain unanswered. The management of pediatric head injury is an area that should be the subject of more clinical trials in the coming years.

There are several obstacles to the organization of more randomized controlled trials in pediatric neurosurgery. For instance, even in the absence of class I data, many pediatric neurosurgical interventions are firmly established as the standard of care for their respective conditions. A trial comparing an accepted surgical therapy with no therapy or another potentially harmful therapy is practically difficult and, in some cases, ethically prohibited. The anxiety that investigators and their institutions may feel about any such studies is invariably heightened when children are the study subjects. Many of the best trials in pediatric neurosurgery have been carried out to investigate new techniques, as in the case of dorsal rhizotomy, or new equipment, as in vagal nerve stimulators or baclofen pumps.

References

1 Drake JM, Kestle JR, Milner R, Cinalli G, Boop F, Piatt J Jr, Haines S, Schiff SJ, Cochrane DD, Steinbok P, MacNeil N: Randomized trial of cerebrospinal fluid shunt valve design in pediatric hydrocephalus. Neurosurgery 1998;43:294–303.

2 Kestle JR, Drake JM, Cochrane DD, Milner R, Walker ML, Abbott R, Boop FA: Lack of benefit of endoscopic ventriculoperitoneal shunt insertion: a multicenter randomized trial. J Neurosurg 2003;98:284–290.

3 Langley JM, LeBlanc JC, Drake J, Milner R: Efficacy of antimicrobial prophylaxis in placement of cerebrospinal fluid shunts: meta-analysis. Clin Infect Dis 1993;17:98–103.

4 Bayston R: Antibiotic prophylaxis in shunt surgery. Dev Med Child Neurol Suppl 1975;35: 99–103.

5 Blomstedt GC: Results of trimethoprim-sulfamethoxazole prophylaxis in ventriculostomy and shunting procedures: a double-blind randomized trial. J Neurosurg 1985;62:694–697.

6 Blum J, Schwartz M, Voth D: Antibiotic single-dose prophylaxis of shunt infections. Neurosurg Rev 1989;12:239–244.

7 Djindjian M, Fevrier MJ, Otterbein G, Soussy JC: Oxacillin prophylaxis in cerebrospinal fluid shunt procedures: results of a randomized open study in 60 hydrocephalic patients. Surg Neurol 1986;25:178–180.

8 Goumnerova L, Hoffman H, Walters B, Humphreys R, Hendrick B: Perioperative antibiotic prophylaxis in shunt surgery (abstract No. 10); in Scientific Program of the Annual Meeting of the American Association of Neurological Surgeons. Washington, American Association of Neurological Surgeons, 1989.

9 Haines SJ, Taylor F: Prophylactic methicillin for shunt operations: effects on incidence of shunt malfunction and infection. Childs Brain 1982;9:10–22.

10 Lambert M, MacKinnon AE, Vaishnav A: Comparison of two methods of prophylaxis against CSF shunt infection. Z Kinderchir 1984;39(suppl 2):109–110.

11 Odio C, Mohs E, Sklar FH, Nelson JD, McCracken GH Jr: Adverse reactions to vancomycin used as prophylaxis for CSF shunt procedures. Am J Dis Child 1984;138:17–19.

12 Reider MJ, Frewen TC, Del Maestro RF, Coyle A, Lovell S: The effect of cephalothin prophylaxis on postoperative ventriculoperitoneal shunt infections. Can Med Assoc J 1987;136:935–938.
13 Schmidt K, Gjerris F, Osgaard O, et al: Antibiotic prophylaxis in cerebrospinal fluid shunting: a prospective randomized trial in 152 hydrocephalic patients. Neurosurgery 1985;17:1–5.
14 Wang EEL, Prober CG, Hendrick BE, Hoffman HJ, Humphreys RP: Prophylactic sulfamethoxazole and trimethoprim in ventriculoperitoneal shunt surgery: a double-blind, randomized, placebo-controlled trial. JAMA 1984;251:1174–1177.
15 Yogev R, Shinco F, McLone D: Prophylaxis for ventriculo-peritoneal shunt surgery with nafcillin alone or in combination with rifampin (abstract No. 664); in Program and Abstracts of the 23rd Interscience Conference on Antimicrobial Agents and Chemotherapy. Washington, American Society for Microbiology, 1983.
16 Walters BC, Goumnerova L, Hoffman HJ, Hendrick EB, Humphreys RP, Levinton C: A randomized controlled trial of perioperative rifampin/trimethoprim in cerebrospinal fluid shunt surgery. Childs Nerv Syst 1992;8:253–257.
16b Zentner J, Gilsbach J, Felder T: Antibiotic prophylaxis in cerebrospinal fluid shunting: a prospective randomized trial in 129 patients. Neurosurg Rev 1995;18:169–172.
17 Govender ST, Nathoo N, Van Dellen JR: Evaluation of an antibiotic-impregnated shunt system for the treatment of hydrocephalus. J Neurosurg 2003;99:831–839.
18 Pfausler B, Spiss H, Beer R, Kampfl A, Engelhardt K, Schober M, Schumutzhard E: Treatment of staphylococcal ventriculitis associated with external cerebrospinal fluid drains: a prospective randomized trial of intravenous compared with intraventricular vancomycin therapy. J Neurosurg 2003;98:1040–1044.
19 Wong GKC, Poon WS, Wai S, Yu LM, Lyon D, Lam JMK: Failure of regular external ventricular drain exchange to reduce cerebrospinal fluid infection: result of a randomized controlled trial. J Neurol Neurosurg Psychiatry 2002;73:759–761.
20 Wiebe S, Blume WT, Girvin JP, Eliasziw M: A randomized, controlled trial of surgery for temporal-lobe epilepsy. N Engl J Med 2001;345:311–318.
21 Engel J, Wiebe S, French J, Sperling M, Williamson P, Spencer D, Gumnit R, Zahn C, Westbrook E, Enos B: Practice parameter: temporal lobe and localized neocortical resections for epilepsy. Neurology 2003;60:538–547.
22 Wyler AR, Hermann BP, Somes G: Extent of medial temporal resection on outcome from anterior temporal lobectomy: a randomized prospective study. Neurosurgery 1995;37:982–990.
23 Ben-Menachem E, Manon-Espaillat R, Ristanovic R, et al: Vagus nerve stimulation for treatment of partial seizures. 1. A controlled study of effect on seizures. Epilepsia 1994;35:614–624.
24 Ramsay RE, Uthman BM, Augustinsson LE, Upton ARM, Naritoku D, Willis J, Treig T, Barolat G, Wernicke JF: Vagus nerve stimulation for treatment of partial seizures. 2. Safety, side effects, and tolerability. Epilepsia 1994;35:627–636.
25 Salinsky MC, Uthman BM, Ristanovic RK, Wernicke JF, Tarver WB; Vagus Nerve Stimulation Study Group: Vagus nerve stimulation for the treatment of medically intractable seizures: results of a 1-year open-extension trial. Arch Neurol 1996;53:1176–1180.
26 Salinsky M, Wernicke JF, Rutecki P, Allen J; The Vagus Nerve Stimulation Study Group: A randomized controlled trial of chronic vagus nerve stimulation for treatment of medically intractable seizures. Neurology 1995;45:224–230.
27 Handforth A, DeGiorgio CM, Schachter SC, et al: Vagus nerve stimulation therapy for partial-onset seizures: a randomized active control trial. Neurology 1998;51:48–55.
28 Grill J, LeDeley M-C, Gambarelli D, Raquin M-A, Couanet D, Pierre-Kahn A, Habrand J-L, Doz F, Frappaz D, Gentet J-C, Edan C, Chastagner P, Kalifa C: Postoperative chemotherapy without irradiation for ependymoma in children under 5 years of age: a multicenter trial of the French Society of Pediatric Oncology. J Clin Oncol 2001;19:1288–1296.
29 Wolff JEA, Gnekow AK, Kortmann R-D, Pietsch T, Urban C, Graf N, Kuhl J: Preradiation chemotherapy for pediatric patients with high-grade glioma. Cancer 2002;94:264–271.
30 Finlay JL, Bayett JM, Yates AJ, et al: Randomized phase III trial in childhood high-grade astrocytoma comparing vincristine, lomustine, and prednisone with eight-drugs-in-1-day regimen. J Clin Oncol 1995;13:112–123.

31 Wisoff JH, Boyett JM, Berger MS, et al: Current neurosurgical management and the impact of the extent of resection in the treatment of malignant gliomas of childhood: a report of the Children's Cancer Group Trial No. CCG-945. J Neurosurg 1998;89:52–59.
32 Kreth FW, Muacevic A: Resection of malignant gliomas of childhood (letter). J Neurosurg 1999;90:1147.
33 Armstrong RW, Steinbok P, Cochrane DD, Kube SD, Fife SE, Farrell K: Intrathecally administered baclofen for treatment of children with spasticity of cerebral origin. J Neurosurg 1997;87: 409–414.
34 Ordia JI, Fischer E, Adamski E: Chronic intrathecal delivery of baclofen by a programmable pump for the treatment of severe spasticity. J Neurosurg 1996;85:452–457.
35 Middel B, Kuipers-Upmeijer H, Bouma J, Staal M, Oenema D, Postma T, Terpstra S, Stewart R: Effect of intrathecal baclofen delivered by an implanted programmable pump on health related quality of life in patients with severe spasticity. J Neurol Neurosurg Psychiatry 1997;63:204–209.
36 McLaughlin JF, Bjornson KF, Astley SJ, Graubert C, Hays RM, Roberts TS, Price R, Temkin N: Selective dorsal rhizotomy: efficacy and safety in an investigator-masked randomized clinical trial. Dev Med Child Neurol 1998;40:220–232.
37 Steinbock P, Reiner AM, Beauchamp R, Armstrong RW, Cochrane DD: A randomized clinical trial to compare selective dorsal rhizotomy plus physiotherapy with physiotherapy alone in children with spastic diplegic cerebral palsy. Dev Med Child Neurol 1997;39:178–184.
38 Wright FV, Sheil EMH, Drake JM, Wedge JH, Naumann S: Evaluation of selective dorsal rhizotomy for the reduction of spasticity in cerebral palsy: a randomized controlled trial. Dev Med Child Neurol 1998;40:239–247.
39 Rosenbaum PL: Selective dorsal rhizotomy studies (letter). Dev Med Child Neurol 1998;40:717.
40 Manning FA, Harrison MR, Rodeck C: Catheter shunts for fetal hydronephrosis and hydrocephalus. N Engl J Med 1986;315:336–340.
41 Farmer DL, von Koch CS, Peacock WJ, Danielpour M, Gupta N, Lee H, Harrison MR: In utero repair of myelomeningocele. Arch Surg 2003;138:872–878.
42 Clewell WH, Johnson ML, Meier PR, Newkirk JB, Zide SL, Hendee RW, Bowes WA Jr, Hecht F, O'Keefe D, Henry GP, Shikes RH: A surgical approach to the treatment of fetal hydrocephalus. N Engl J Med 1982;306:1320–1325.
43 Michejda M, Queenan JT, McCullough D: Present status of intrauterine treatment of hydrocephalus and its future. Am J Obstet Gynecol 1986;155:873–882.
44 Sutton LN, Adzick NS, Johnson MP: Fetal surgery for myelomenigocele. Childs Nerv Syst 2003;19:587–591.
45 Young KD, Okada PJ, Sokolove PE, Palchak MJ, Panacek EA, Baren JM, Huff KR, McBride DQ, Inkelis SH, Lewis RJ: A randomized, double-blinded, placebo-controlled trial of phenytoin for the prevention of early posttraumatic seizures in children with moderate to severe blunt head injury. Ann Emerg Med 2004;43:435–446.
46 Taylor A, Butt W, Rosenfeld J, Shann F, Ditchfield M, Lewis E, Klug G, Wallace D, Henning R, Tibballs J: A randomized trial of very early decompressive craniectomy in children with traumatic brain injury and sustained intracranial hypertension. Childs Nerv Syst 2001;17:154–162.

Corey Raffel, MD, PhD
Mayo Clinic, 200 First St., SW
Rochester, MN 55905 (USA)
Tel. +1 507 284 8167, E-Mail raffel.corey@mayo.edu

Pollock BE (ed): Guiding Neurosurgery by Evidence.
Prog Neurol Surg. Basel, Karger, 2006, vol 19, pp 107–122

Cerebrovascular-Endovascular

Kevin M. Cockroft[a], *Robert H. Rosenwasser*[b]

[a]Department of Neurosurgery, Penn State Hershey Medical Center, Hershey, Pa.,
[b]Department of Neurological Surgery, Thomas Jefferson University Hospital, Philadelphia, Pa., USA

Abstract

This chapter will review the current status of scientific knowledge to support evidence-based medicine guidelines for the endovascular treatment of cerebrovascular disease. Three major areas of cerebrovascular disease will be examined, (1) occlusive cerebrovascular disease, (2) vascular malformations and (3) intracranial aneurysms. Levels of evidence vary in each area and the reasons for this variation as well as the challenges that may limit further investigations are discussed.

As a relatively new area of subspecialization within neurosurgery, endovascular neurosurgery represents an area ripe for scientific investigation. However, while numerous questions within the field remain unanswered, several obstacles exist that may prevent many investigations from ever reaching fruition. As with 'open' cerebrovascular surgery, endovascular neurosurgery involves three major disease categories: (1) occlusive cerebrovascular disease, (2) vascular malformations and (3) intracranial aneurysms. Within each group there are varying degrees of scientific data to support evidence-based medicine guidelines. This chapter will consider the current state of evidence-based medicine in each of these three areas and then examine some of the issues and limitations facing further scientific study in these areas.

Occlusive Cerebrovascular Disease: Carotid Artery Stenosis

The mainstay of the open surgical treatment of occlusive cerebrovascular disease, the carotid endarterectomy (CEA), may arguably be the most

Table 1. Comparison of major prospective randomized trials comparing CEA with CAS [adapted from 77]

Study name	Date published	Patients, n		Stroke or death within 30 days, n		
		endovascular	surgical	endovascular	surgical	odds ratio (95% CI)
SAPPHIRE[a]	2002	156	151	7 (4.5)	10 (6.6)	0.87 (0.25–1.77)
CAVATAS[b]	2001	251	253	25 (10.0)	25 (10.0)	1.01 (0.56–1.81)
Kentucky[c]	2001	53	51	0	1 (2.0)	0.13 (0.00–6.56)
Leicester[d]	1998	11	12	5 (45.4)	0	12.88 (1.85–89.61)

Figures in parentheses represent percentage or 95% CI.

[a]Stenting and Angioplasty with Protection in Patients at High Risk for Endarterectomy trial [12] not published in a peer-reviewed format.

[b]Carotid and Vertebral Artery Transluminal Angioplasty Study [10].

[c]CAS versus CEA for treatment of asymptomatic carotid stenosis: a randomized trial in a community hospital [78].

[d]Randomized study of CAS versus CEA: a stopped trial [9].

comprehensively studied of all neurosurgical procedures. To a large degree this befits the role of CEA as the most common surgical procedure performed for stroke, the number three cause of mortality in the United States and the leading cause of disability in US adults. In contrast, the endovascular counterpart to CEA, carotid angioplasty and stenting (CAS) is much less well studied (table 1). To date much of the literature on the efficacy of CAS comes mostly from uncontrolled case series and registry data [1–8].

The results of the first attempt at a randomized clinical trial comparing CEA and CAS were published in 1998 [9]. This trial, performed at a single center in the United Kingdom, was stopped prematurely after 5 of the first 7 patients undergoing CAS had a stroke (3 of which were disabling at 30 days). This early study did not utilize distal protection devices during CAS and since its publication numerous case series and registry results have been published both with and without distal protection, suggesting more reasonable rates of stroke and death. A subsequent randomized multicenter trial performed in Europe, Australia and Canada, the Carotid and Vertebral Artery Transluminal Angioplasty Study (CAVATAS), showed similar rates of stroke and death at 30 days for both CEA and CAS [10]. However, the overall complication rate for both procedures was 10%. This percentage appears high when compared to previously published CEA data and is higher than American Heart Association (AHA) guidelines for symptomatic carotid stenosis, which suggest that the combined morbidity and mortality from surgery should not exceed 6% [11].

More recent work using distal protection during CAS has yielded more favorable results. In the Carotid Revascularization using Endarterectomy or Stenting Systems (CARESS) trial, a multicenter phase I trial comparing CAS with distal protection and CEA, 397 patients were treated, 254 with CEA and 143 with CAS. Baseline characteristics between the two groups were similar except that CAS patients were almost 3 times as likely to have undergone a previous CEA as compared to patients in the CEA group. A history of a previous carotid stent was also more common in the CAS group. In the end there was no significant difference in the 30-day rates of stroke and all-cause mortality between the two groups, suggesting that CAS may be appropriate in patients with a previous history of a carotid artery procedure.

Although as yet not published in a peer-reviewed format, the results of the SAPPHIRE (Stenting and Angioplasty with Protection in Patients at High Risk for Endarterectomy) trial, an industry-sponsored prospective randomized trial, has lent support to the concept that CAS may be better than CEA for 'high-risk' patients [12]. In this trial's cohort of mostly asymptomatic patients, the 30-day risk of stroke, myocardial infarction (MI) and death was 3.8, 2.6 and 0.6%, respectively, in the CAS group and 5.3, 7.3 and 2.0% in the CEA group. When assessed separately, none of the differences in these individual results reached statistical significance. However, when combined into a single endpoint, analysis yielded a significantly reduced adverse event risk for CAS as compared to CEA. Obviously the major factor in this difference is the rate of MI, which turns out to be largely made up of subendocardial (non-Q wave) infarctions. Whether such 'chemical MIs' are in fact clinically significant or simply markers of high cardiac risk status remains controversial. Questions have also been raised as to the appropriateness of the high-risk criteria used. One Mayo Clinic retrospective review of 323 CEA patients, selected based on the SAPPHIRE high-risk criteria, reported overall rates of stroke, MI and death as 1.65, 0.83 and 1.65%, respectively, rates which were not much different to SAPPHIRE's CAS group [13]. In addition, it has been argued that the use of regional anesthesia reduces the risk of cardiopulmonary morbidity and mortality after CEA in 'high-risk' patients [14–16], thus bringing the overall risk of CEA in high-risk patients in line with that of CAS in the SAPPHIRE trial.

While controversy still exists regarding the indications for CAS, technological advances and early trial results are leading to an increased acceptance of distal protection devices. During the early stages of the Endarterectomy versus Angioplasty in Patients with Symptomatic Severe Carotid Stenosis (EVA-3S) trial, an analysis of the first 80 patients randomized to CAS prompted the trial's data safety monitoring committee to recommend stopping the performance of unprotected CAS after an almost 4-fold increase in the 30-day stroke rate was found in the unprotected CAS group as compared to the protected CAS patients

[17]. All current CAS trials now include the use of a distal protection device, either as an option or a requirement.

At this point there is no class I evidence to suggest that CAS is a better alternative to CEA in either asymptomatic patients or symptomatic patients that are eligible for CEA. The preponderance of evidence would seem to suggest that CAS may be a lower risk than CEA in patients with medical contraindications to surgical endarterectomy or with local surgical risk factors such as postradiation-induced stenosis, history of prior CEA and/or a high bifurcation. From a scientific standpoint, the inability to consistently demonstrate a significant difference (or even equivalence) between the two methods of treatment, the heterogeneity of previous studies and the evolution of angioplasty/stent technology certainly support further prospective randomized trials. However, market forces and public perceptions are rapidly shaping clinical practice to the point that these ongoing studies may be in jeopardy of failing to meet recruitment goals. As such the strongest indication for CAS at the present time, may as part of a randomized clinical trial such as CREST in the US, CAVATAS II in the UK, EVA-3S in France or SPACE (Stent Protected Angioplasty versus Carotid Endarterectomy) in Germany.

Occlusive Cerebrovascular Disease: Acute Stroke

Based largely on the 1995 publication of the National Institute of Neurological Disorders and Stroke (NINDS) study of intravenous (IV) thrombolysis for acute ischemic stroke and the subsequent Food and Drug Administration (FDA) approval of recombinant tissue plasminogen activator (rt-PA) for this indication, AHA guidelines now suggest that patients with a defined stroke onset of within 3 h should be considered for IV rt-PA [18]. Since the NINDS study established a 3-hour time period for efficacy with IV rt-PA, various attempts have been made to extend this therapeutic window by demonstrating efficacy for IV thrombolysis up to 6 h after the onset of ischemia.

While data supporting the extension of the therapeutic window for IV thrombolysis have been mixed, evidence mainly from the Prolyse in Acute Cerebral Thromboembolism (PROACT) studies suggests that intra-arterial (IA) thrombolysis may be beneficial up to 6 h after the onset of ischemia. The initial PROACT study published in 1998 randomized 49 patients with early middle cerebral artery (MCA) territory ischemia to either IA recombinant prourokinase (r-proUK) or placebo [19]. The recanalization rate, the primary endpoint, was significantly higher in the r-proUK group as compared to the placebo-treated group. The r-proUK group also demonstrated a reduction in 90-day mortality from 43 to 27%, although the small number of patients in the study prevented this difference from reaching statistical significance. Not unexpectedly, there was a higher incidence of hemorrhagic transformation in the r-proUK group, 15 versus 7%. However, this difference was also not statistically significant. PROACT II, involving 180 patients from 54 centers and published the following year, did demonstrate a significant improvement in outcome at 90 days for patients treated with r-proUK and heparin as compared to those treated with heparin alone [20]. Recanalization rates remained significantly better for r-proUK treated patients, although overall mortality was similar. Again intracerebral hemorrhage was more common in the treatment group, but this difference was still not statistically significant. In the vertebrobasilar system, acute thromboocclusive disease carries a particularly poor prognosis. Although not as extensively studied, results from case series of IA thrombolysis in the posterior circulation have been promising and appear to suggest an even larger therapeutic window [21, 22].

Various means of mechanical thrombolysis have been tried in an effort to promote improved clot disruption while minimizing the dose of thrombolytic agent and thereby hopefully reducing the rate of secondary hemorrhage [23–28]. The recently published results of the Mechanical Embolus Removal in Cerebral Ischemia (MERCI) study [29] have also been encouraging in this regard. The study was a phase I device trial for the Merci Retrieval System, a corkscrew-like device designed for mechanical embolectomy in the cerebral vasculature. Successful recanalization with the device alone was achieved in 12 of 28 patients (43%) and with the addition of IA rt-PA in 18 patients (64%). There were 12 asymptomatic and no symptomatic intracranial hemorrhages. Only one procedure-related technical complication occurred and this was of no clinical consequence. The device is now FDA approved and a registry of post-approval patients will be maintained.

In addition to IA thrombolysis in the acute phase of stroke, other endovascular techniques, namely intracranial angioplasty and/or stenting, are becoming increasingly popular as preventative treatments. Relatively high rates of technical success in patients with refractory symptomatic intracranial atherosclerotic disease have been reported [30–35]. Improved clinical outcome, on the other hand, has been less frequent and complications have been problematic. In the vertebrobasilar circulation in particular, complication rates as high as 25–38% have been published [22, 36–39]. Although promising, at this point more research is still needed to clarify the efficacy of intracranial angioplasty/stenting in stroke prevention for patients with persistent ischemic symptoms secondary to atherosclerotic disease in the cerebral circulation.

Current clinical research in acute stroke continues to focus on methods of extending the therapeutic window for thrombolysis, either with IV or IA administration alone or in combination. The Emergency Management of Stroke

(EMS) Bridging Trial, a pilot, placebo-controlled multicenter study randomized 35 patients to IV and IA rt-PA, or placebo and IA rt-PA within 3 h [40]. The study demonstrated improved recanalization in the IV/IA group as compared to the placebo/IA group. The numbers of intracerebral hemorrhages were similar in the two groups. As a phase I study the trial was underpowered to detect efficacy and no statistically significant difference in clinical outcome was seen between the two groups. Further studies are underway to better assess the safety and efficacy of such 'bridging' regimens.

At present, the existing evidence suggests that IA thrombolysis (rt-PA or urokinase) may be indicated in patients with signs and symptoms of cerebral ischemia and large intracranial vessel occlusion within 6 h of symptom onset. Mechanical clot disruption/retrieval may be a useful adjunct to chemical thrombolysis in select patients and may be a reasonable alternative in other patients who are ineligible for chemical thrombolysis or who fall just outside the 6-hour treatment window.

Vascular Malformations

For the most part endovascular embolization is employed as an adjunctive therapy in the treatment of CNS vascular malformations. For the purposes of this chapter we will examine the evidence for the endovascular embolization of cerebral (pial) AVMs either for cure or as an adjunct to microsurgical resection or stereotactic radiosurgery.

While microsurgical removal may provide an immediate cure for accessible lesions, resection of malformations with a large nidus, deep feeding vessels, and/or high-flow shunts may carry a relatively high risk of morbidity. In such patients, it is theorized that the added benefits of endovascular treatment outweigh the small additional risks and compare favorably with the risks of surgery alone. This conclusion stems largely from a variety of nonrandomized, mostly retrospective case series, the results of which have shown improved outcomes, shortened operative time and reduced blood loss in patients with preoperative embolization as compared to patients with microsurgical resection alone [41–49].

The largest prospective randomized controlled trial to assess endovascular embolization of AVMs was actually an industry-sponsored equivalency trial designed to support FDA approval for N-butyl cyanoacrylate (NBCA) in the treatment of intracranial AVMs. Published in 2002, the study compared NBCA with the then 'standard of care' polyvinyl alcohol (PVA) particles for the preoperative embolization of cerebral AVMs. The study demonstrated equivalence for both agents, at least in terms of the percentage of nidus reduction and number of pedicles embolized [50]. Interestingly, many centers that commonly used 'glue' to embolize AVMs as an 'off-label' indication were so convinced of its superiority that they did not take part in the study because participating patients would have to be randomized. This problem of investigator bias is commonplace in clinical trials and in some instances may result in insufficient scientific evidence ever being generated to support a product or device use. In the case of NBCA, however, equivalency was enough to allow for FDA approval and clinical practice combined with market forces have led NBCA embolization to almost completely supplant PVA embolization for cerebral AVMs.

The majority of studies would suggest that cerebral/pial AVMs are rarely cured by endovascular embolization alone and there are no prospective randomized studies comparing cure and complication rates for surgical resection versus endovascular embolization for AVMs amenable to either treatment. Making a judgment based on 'cure rates' from published series is probably inappropriate. Since embolization evolved primarily as a therapeutic adjunct, many published series suffer from considerable referral bias, whereby only 'large' AVMs incapable of being treated with radiosurgery or open microsurgery alone are referred for embolization and smaller lesions with only one or two feeding pedicles are treated without endovascular intervention. In addition, the lack of a widely accepted endovascular grading scale makes comparison between various studies problematic. In general, most studies of intracranial AVMs, not specifically selected for endovascular treatment alone, report cure rates with embolization of between 5 and 10% [44, 47, 51, 52]. Gobin et al. [53] found a cure rate of 11.2% in a cohort of 125 patients scheduled for radiosurgery who had undergone embolization initially as an 'adjunctive' therapy. In contrast, other authors have reported much higher rates of cure with endovascular therapy when patients were selected specifically for embolization as a primary modality. After selecting a subgroup of patients on the basis of angiographic features that they felt were likely to promote endovascular obliteration, Valavanis and Yasargil [54] noted a cure rate of 74% (or 35% of their overall series) with embolization alone. Of course none of these studies included a contemporaneous control group, much less prospective randomization.

Endovascular embolization is also commonly used as an adjunct to stereotactic radiosurgery. In patients with AVMs located in eloquent cortex or deep structures, stereotactic radiosurgery may be a preferable alternative to microsurgical resection where the risk of morbidity and mortality may be unacceptably high. In such patients, endovascular embolization may be employed to reduce the size of the AVM prior to radiosurgery or to eliminate certain angiographic features, such as intranidal aneurysms, that may provide an elevated risk while the patient is awaiting AVM obliteration after radiosurgery.

It is well known that the rate of AVM cure after stereotactic radiosurgery decreases as the volume of the AVM being treated increases [55–62]. Case series have shown higher cure rates for patients undergoing radiosurgical treatment with AVM volumes below 10 cm^3 or average diameter less than 3 cm [53, 60, 63]. Therefore, the role of endovascular embolization in this setting is to reduce the nidus size, such that a cure after radiosurgery will be more likely [56, 58, 64]. This view is, however, somewhat controversial and, although less of a problem with NBCA, some centers have reported apparent recanalization of previously embolized portions of AVM [60, 63, 65]. For those patients in whom the lesion does not proceed to obliteration after stereotactic radiosurgery, repeated embolization or surgical resection may still be employed, often with greater success [66, 67].

Although only complete elimination of the AVM constitutes a true cure, palliative treatment may be employed in selected cases. Specifically, patients who are symptomatic with large and/or deep-seated AVMs that are unlikely to be cured with any combination of modalities may benefit from subtotal endovascular embolization. In patients with repeated hemorrhages, embolization may be used to eliminate angiographic risk factors for hemorrhage, such as intranidal aneurysms. For those with intractable headaches or progressive neurological deficits, the benefits of partial treatment are less certain. Nonetheless, embolization to reduce the arteriovenous shunt, and thereby decrease the amount of 'steal' and/or venous hypertension associated with a lesion, has been reported to cause clinical improvement [68, 69]. Overall, though, the concept that partial treatment of an AVM is at all beneficial is still controversial, and a similar or worse natural history in incompletely treated patients has certainly been reported [70, 71].

In summary, there is class I evidence to suggest that preoperative glue embolization with NBCA is equivalent to PVA embolization for cerebral AVMs and there is class II evidence supporting a role for glue embolization as an adjunct to microsurgical and radiosurgical treatment of pial AVMs. Evidence for endovascular embolization as a palliative treatment for pial AVMs is minimal and inconsistent. Given the current widespread use of NBCA and in-grained patterns of multimodality treatment, it is unlikely that another prospective randomized trial, this time designed to show efficacy for embolization (adjunctive or otherwise) over microsurgical or radiosurgical treatment alone, will ever be performed.

Endovascular Aneurysm Coiling

Perhaps the most controversial recent development in cerebrovascular neurosurgery has been the introduction and swift progression to widespread use of the Guglielmi Detachable Coil (GDC) for the treatment of intracranial aneurysms. Originally approved by the FDA in 1991 under an Investigational Device Exemption (IDE), over 250,000 patients worldwide have now been

Table 2. Summary of results from International Subarachnoid Aneurysm Trial (ISAT) [72], 9,559 patients assessed for eligibility and 2,143 patients (22%) randomized

Treatment group	Patients, n	1-year rebleed rate[a] %	Dead or dependent at 2 months[b], n	Dead or dependent at 1 year[b], n
Microsurgical clipping	1,070	0.9 (26)	345 (36.4)	243 (30.6)
Endovascular coiling	1,073	2.7 (66)	244 (25.4)*	190 (23.7)*

*Statistically significant values.
[a]Figures in parentheses represent number of patients.
[b]Figures in parentheses represent percentage.

treated with GDC and the technology has spawned a host of imitators. The initial clinical trial that led to FDA approval focused on patients with 'inoperable or high-risk aneurysms' and in the first few years after approval, posterior circulation and other surgically challenging aneurysms were the most common types of intracranial aneurysms treated with endovascular techniques. However, this distribution of cases has been rapidly changing. To a large degree market forces, including widespread access to healthcare information via the Internet, aggressive marketing by various manufacturers and consumer (patient) choice, have driven this evolution. However, class I clinical evidence has also been forthcoming to support the use of endovascular coiling, at least in ruptured intracranial aneurysms.

The study that has had the most impact in this direction is the International Subarachnoid Aneurysm Trial (ISAT) [72]. Published in October 2002 in *Lancet*, this prospective randomized trial compared neurosurgical clipping with endovascular coiling in 2,143 patients with ruptured intracranial aneurysms. The results demonstrated an advantage for endovascular coiling over surgical clipping at 1 year. Specifically, in patients with ruptured intracranial aneurysms for whom endovascular coiling and microsurgical clipping are therapeutic options, the outcome in terms of survival, free of disability at 1 year was significantly better with endovascular coiling as compared to microsurgical clipping (table 2). This landmark study deserves some further comment.

A total of 9,559 patients were assessed for study eligibility, of these 2,143 (22%) were randomized. The randomized patients were evenly distributed between the endovascular group (1,073 patients) and the neurosurgical group (1,070 patients). Age, sex and neurological grade were evenly distributed. The time between subarachnoid hemorrhage and randomization was virtually identical in both groups. Over 95% of the aneurysms randomized were in the anterior circulation, with the majority of these being in the anterior cerebral artery distribution (50%). Only 14% were located in the MCA distribution, and only 2.7% were in the posterior circulation. Nonprocedural bleeding from the target aneurysm was higher in the neurosurgical group, where 23 patients bled prior to a definitive surgical management as compared to 14 in the endovascular group. An assessment of clinical outcome in 1,906 patients at 2 months revealed that 25.4% of patients were dead or dependent in the endovascular group compared to 36.4% in the neurosurgical group ($p < 0.0001$). At 1 year, data from 1,594 patients demonstrated a 23.7% rate of death and disability in the endovascular group versus a rate of 30.6% in the neurosurgical group ($p = 0.0019$). This difference represents an approximately 22% relative-risk reduction or an absolute-risk reduction of 6.9% for endovascular treatment over microsurgical clipping at 1 year.

This 22% reduction in the *relative* risk was widely reported in the popular press and has contributed in no small way to the increased popularity of endovascular techniques for the treatment of intracranial aneurysms. However, from a scientific point of view there are several features of this trial, which should preclude the generalization of its findings to the treatment of all intracranial aneurysms, both ruptured and unruptured. Most importantly, the patients enrolled in ISAT do not constitute a random sample of patients with intracranial aneurysms. Rather these patients were selected from among patients with a subarachnoid hemorrhage and an intracranial aneurysm that was felt by the treating physicians to be equally amenable to either microsurgical clipping or endovascular coiling. MCA aneurysms were underrepresented as the consensus among most practitioners continues to be that these are difficult to successfully treat by endovascular means. Similarly, posterior circulation aneurysms, heavily represented in the initial trial for the FDA approval of GDC, are now almost exclusively treated by endovascular means and as such even fewer posterior circulation aneurysms were randomized.

Interestingly, at 1 year, some secondary endpoints actually favored surgery, posttreatment rebleeding was 2.9 times more likely in the endovascular group, death was 2.8 times more likely in the endovascular group and endovascular patients were 4 times more likely to require additional treatment. In addition, 1-year case-fatality rates were not significantly different. However, the primary endpoint of death and disability included all these parameters and showed an overall benefit to endovascular therapy.

ISAT has also been criticized on a variety of other levels. The fact that only 2,143 (22%) of a total of 9,559 screened patients were randomized and the finding that the majority of those not randomized underwent surgical treatment for their aneurysm have led some to speculate on a systemic selection bias. The study participants are primarily European, with a handful of Canadian groups and only one US center. This distribution of study centers, combined with memories of the International Cooperative Study [73] where early surgery after aneurysmal subarachnoid hemorrhage improved outcome in North America but not in Europe, has prompted concerns over the generalizability of the study's results to North American patients. The relatively high 1-year rebleed rate in the surgical group (0.9% as compared to 2.7% in the GDC group) has also raised concerns, as this surgical rebleed rate does not appear to reflect the North American experience. In addition, ISAT has been criticized for the lack of adjudication of the participating neurosurgeons' operative experience, including perioperative morbidity and mortality. Some of the surgeons who participated in the trial had clipped fewer than 10 aneurysms per year. Also of concern, the major finding of ISAT is only statistically significant when the primary outcome of death and disability is defined as a modified Rankin Score (mRS) 3–6. If mRS 2 ('some restriction in lifestyle') is included in the disabled group or if mRS 3 ('significant lifestyle restriction') is removed from the disability group, then the difference in the primary outcome between the endovascular and surgical groups is no longer statistically significant. Finally, since previous case series have shown relatively high rates of aneurysm recurrence after coiling, the use of a 1-year outcome has been criticized as inappropriately short.

Criticism aside, to date ISAT provides the best class I evidence comparing endovascular coiling with microsurgical clipping for ruptured intracranial aneurysms. The trial outcome supports the conclusion that endovascular treatment for selected patients with ruptured aneurysms may yield a better outcome than surgical treatment, at least at 1 year. Although not specifically looked at in the first ISAT report, various other nonrandomized cohort studies have reported a shorter length of stay and lower hospital charges for patients with aneurysms treated with endovascular coiling as opposed to surgical clipping [74–76]. These same studies have also shown comparatively better outcomes in patients with *unruptured* aneurysms treated by endovascular methods.

Efforts to resolve some of the controversial issues raised by ISAT and other retrospective studies have led to the consideration of a North American trial. The North American Trial for Unruptured and Ruptured Aneurysms (NATURE), supported by both the American Association of Neurological Surgeons and the Congress of Neurological Surgeons is being considered for funding by the National Institutes of Health. However, the final status of such a trial is still uncertain. As with NBCA glue embolization, the widespread use of endovascular coiling, combined with the already well-established treatment patterns for certain aneurysms as well as the strongly held beliefs of many practitioners and patients, will likely preclude randomization of *all* types of intracranial aneurysms and may hamper recruitment even in a trial of more limited scope.

Conclusions

Endovascular neurosurgery continues to be a field in the midst of rapid growth and development. As the indications for endovascular treatment expand, new devices become available and existing therapies improve; the need for good clinical evidence to support treatment decisions will be as important as ever. However, as we have seen the reasons why medical evidence exists or does not exist for certain procedures are extensive and complex. As medicine becomes increasingly driven by technology and that technology is marketed directly to patients and supplied by industry rather than by academic or governmental developments, it may become increasingly difficult to obtain class I evidence for a given procedure or treatment. In many instances, clinicians and consumers alike will be left to base their management decisions on the careful evaluation of uncontrolled case series, retrospective cohort studies or industry-sponsored equivalency trials.

References

1 Yadav JS, Roubin GS, Iyer SJ, Vitek J, King P, Jordan WD, Fisher WS: Elective stenting of the extracranial carotid arteries. Circulation 1997;95:376–381.

2 Roubin GS, Yadav JS, Iyer SS, Vitek JJ: Carotid stent-supported angioplasty: neurovascular intervention to prevent stroke. Am J Cardiol 1996;78:8–12.

3 Iyer SS, Roubin GS, Yadav JS, Diethrich EB, Whorley MH, Shawl FA: Angioplasty and stenting for extracranial carotid stenosis: multicenter experience. Circulation 1996;94:1–58.

4 Theron JG, Payelle GG, Coskun O, Huet JF, Guimaraens L: Carotid artery stenosis treatment with protected balloon angioplasty and stent placement. Radiology 1996;201:627–636.

5 Vozzi CR, Rodriguez AO, Paolantonio D, Smith JA, Wholey MH: Extracranial carotid angioplasty and stenting: initial results and short-term follow-up. Tex Heart Inst J 1997;24:167–172.

6 Iyer SS, Roubin GS, Yadav JS, Vitek J, Parks JA, Wadlington V: Elective carotid stenting. J Endovasc Surg 1996;3:105–106.

7 Kachel R: Results of balloon angioplasty in carotid arteries. J Endovasc Surg 1996;3:22–30.

8 Qureshi AI, Fareed M, Suri K, Wadsworth DC, Dulin J, Hopkins LN: Multicenter study of the feasibility and safety of using the Memotherm carotid arterial stent for extracranial carotid artery stenosis. J Neurosurg 2002;96:830–836.

9 Naylor AR, Bolia A, Abbot R, Pye IF, Smith J, Lennard N, Lloyd AJ, London NJM, Bell PRF: Randomized study of carotid angioplasty and stenting versus carotid endarterectomy: a stopped trial. J Vasc Surg 1998;28:326–334.

10 Endovascular versus surgical treatment in patients with carotid stenosis in the Carotid and Vertebral Artery Transluminal Angioplasty Study (CAVATAS): a randomized trial. Lancet 2001;357:1729–1737.

11 Biller J, Feinberg WM, Castaldo JE, Whittemore AD, Harbaugh RE, Dempsey RJ, Caplan LR, Kresowik TF, Matchar DB, Toole J, Easton JD, Adams HP, Brass LM, Hobson R, Brott T, Sternau L: Guidelines for carotid endarterectomy: a statement for healthcare professionals from a special writing group of the Stroke Council, American Heart Association. Stroke 1998;29: 554–562.

12 Yadav JS: Stenting and angioplasty with protection in patients at high risk for endarterectomy (SAPPHIRE study). American Heart Association Scientific Sessions, Chicago, Nov 19, 2002.

13 Mozes G, Sullivan TM, Torres-Russoto DR, Bower TC, Hoskin TL, Sampaio SM, Gloviczki P, Panneton JM, Noel AA, Cherry KJ: Carotid endarterectomy in SAPPHIRE-eligible high-risk patients: implications for selecting patients for carotid angioplasty and stenting. J Vasc Surg 2004;39:958–965.
14 Sbarigia E, Dario Vizza C, Antonini M, Speziale F, Maritti M, Fiorani B, Fedele F: Locoregional versus general anesthesia in carotid surgery: is there an impact on perioperative myocardial ischemia? Results of a prospective monocentric randomized trial. J Vasc Surg 1999;30: 131–138.
15 Harbaugh RE, Magnadottir HB: Carotid endarterectomy in high risk patients. Neurol Res 2002;24:S66–70.
16 Magnadottir HB, Lightdale N, Harbaugh RE: Clinical outcome for patients at high risk who underwent carotid endarterectomy with regional anesthesia. Neurosurgery 1999;45:786–791.
17 Mas JL, Chatellier G, Beyssen B: Carotid angioplasty and stenting with and without cerebral protection: clinical alert from the Endarterectomy versus Angioplasty in Patients with Symptomatic Severe Carotid Stenosis (EVA-3S) trial. Stroke 2004;35:e18–20.
18 Tissue plasminogen activator for acute ischemic stroke. The National Institute of Neurological Disorders and Stroke rt-PA Stroke Study Group. N Engl J Med 1995;333:1581–1587.
19 del Zoppo GJ, Higashida RT, Furlan AJ, Pessin MS, Rowley HA, Gent M: PROACT: a phase II randomized trial of recombinant pro-urokinase by direct arterial delivery in acute middle cerebral artery stroke. PROACT Investigators. Prolyse in Acute Cerebral Thromboembolism. Stroke 1998;29:1255–1256.
20 Furlan AJ, Higashida RT, Wechsler LR, Gent M, Rowley HA, Kase C, Pessin MS, Ahuja A, Callahan F, Clark WM, Silver F, Rivera F: Intra-arterial prourokinase for acute ischemic stroke. The PROACT II study: a randomized controlled trial. Prolyse in Acute Cerebral Thromboembolism. JAMA 1999;282:2003–2011.
21 Schellinger PD, Fiebach JB, Mohr A, Ringleb PA, Jansen O, Hacke W: Thrombolytic therapy for ischemic stroke – a review. II. Intra-arterial thrombolysis, vertebrobasilar stroke, phase IV trials, and stroke imaging. Crit Care Med 2001;29:1819–1825.
22 Wijdicks EF, Nichols DA, Thielen KR, Fulgham JR, Brown RD, Meissner I, Meyer FB, Piepgras DG: Intra-arterial thrombolysis in acute basilar artery thromboembolism: the initial Mayo Clinic experience. Mayo Clin Proc 1997;72:1005–1013.
23 Berlis A, Lutsep H, Barnwell S, Norbash A, Wechsler L, Jungreis CA, Woolfenden A, Redekop G, Hartmann M, Schumacher M: Mechanical thrombolysis in acute ischemic stroke with endovascular photoacoustic recanalization. Stroke 2004;35:1112–1126.
24 Sorimachi T, Fujii Y, Tsuchiya N, Nashimoto T, Harada A, Ito Y, Tanaka R: Recanalization by mechanical embolus disruption during intra-arterial thrombolysis in the carotid territory. AJNR Am J Neuroradiol 2004;25:1391–1402.
25 Daffertshofer M, Hennerici M: Ultrasound in the treatment of ischaemic stroke. Lancet Neurol 2003;2:283–290.
26 Kerber CW, Barr JD, Berger RM, Chopko BW: Snare retrieval of intracranial thrombus in patients with acute stroke. J Vasc Interv Radiol 2002;13:1269–1274.
27 Qureshi AI, Siddiqui AM, Suri MF, Kim SH, Ali Z, Yahia AM, Lopes DK, Boulos AS, Ringer AJ, Saad M, Guterman LR, Hopkins LN: Aggressive mechanical clot disruption and low-dose intra-arterial third-generation thrombolytic agent for ischemic stroke: a prospective study. Neurosurgery 2002;51:1319–1329.
28 Ringer AJ, Qureshi AI, Fessler RD, Guterman LR, Hopkins LN: Angioplasty of intracranial occlusion resistant to thrombolysis in acute ischemic stroke. Neurosurgery 2001;48:1282–1288.
29 Gobin YP, Starkman S, Duckwiler GR, Grobelny T, Kidwell CS, Jahan R, Pile-Spellman J, Segal A, Vinuela F, Saver JL: MERCI 1: a phase 1 study of mechanical embolus removal in cerebral ischemia. Stroke 2004;35:2848–2854.
30 Lee TH, Kim DH, Lee BH, Kim HJ, Choi CH, Park KP, Jung DS, Kim S, Moon TY: Preliminary results of endovascular stent-assisted angioplasty for symptomatic middle cerebral artery stenosis. AJNR Am J Neuroradiol 2005;26:166–174.
31 de Rochemont Rdu M, Turowski B, Buchkremer M, Sitzer M, Zanella FE, Berkefeld J: Recurrent symptomatic high-grade intracranial stenoses: safety and efficacy of undersized stents – initial experience. Radiology 2004;231:45–49.

32 Kim JK, Ahn JY, Lee BH, Chung YS, Chung SS, Kim OJ, Kim WC, Joo JY: Elective stenting for symptomatic middle cerebral artery stenosis presenting as transient ischaemic deficits or stroke attacks: short term arteriographical and clinical outcome. J Neurol Neurosurg Psychiatry 2004;75: 847–851.

33 Lee JH, Kwon SU, Lee JH, Suh DC, Kim JS: Percutaneous transluminal angioplasty for symptomatic middle cerebral artery stenosis: long-term follow-up. Cerebrovasc Dis 2003;15:90–97.

34 Alazzaz A, Thornton J, Aletich V, Debrun G, Ausman J, Charbel F: Intracranial percutaneous transluminal angioplasty for arteriosclerotic stenosis. Arch Neurol 2000;57:1625–1630.

35 Marks MP, Marcellus M, Norbash AM, Steinberg GK, Tong D, Albers GW: Outcome of angioplasty for atherosclerotic intracranial stenosis. Stroke 1999;30:1065–1069.

36 Gress DR, Smith WS, Dowd CF, Van Halbach V, Finley RJ, Higashida RT: Angioplasty for intracranial symptomatic vertebrobasilar ischemia. Neurosurgery 2002;51:23–27.

37 Levy EI, Horowitz MB, Koebbe CJ, Jungreis CC, Pride GL, Dutton K, Purdy PD: Transluminal stent-assisted angioplasty of the intracranial vertebrobasilar system for medically refractory, posterior circulation ischemia: early results. Neurosurgery 2001;48:1215–1221.

38 Levy EI, Hanel RA, Bendok BR, Boulos AS, Hartney ML, Guterman LR, Qureshi AI, Hopkins LN: Staged stent-assisted angioplasty for symptomatic intracranial vertebrobasilar artery stenosis. J Neurosurg 2002;97:1294–1301.

39 Rasmussen PA, Perl J, Barr JD, Markarian GZ, Katzan I, Sila C: Stent-assisted angioplasty of intracranial vertebrobasilar atherosclerosis: an initial experience. J Neurosurg 2000;92:771–778.

40 Lewandowski CA, Frankel M, Tomsick TA, Broderick J, Frey J, Clark W, Starkman S, Grotta J, Spilker J, Khoury J, Brott T: Combined intravenous and intra-arterial r-TPA versus intra-arterial therapy of acute ischemic stroke: Emergency Management of Stroke (EMS) Bridging Trial. Stroke 1999;30:2598–2605.

41 Jafar JJ, David AJ, Berenstein A, Choi IS, Kupersmith MJ: The effect of embolization with N-butyl-cyanoacrylate prior to surgical resection of cerebral arteriovenous malformations. J Neurosurg 1993;78:60–69.

42 Spetzler RF, Martin NA, Carter LP, Flom RA, Raudzens PA, Wilkinson E: Surgical management of large AVM's by staged embolization and operative excision. J Neurosurg 1987;67:17–28.

43 Pasqualin A, Scienza R, Cioffi F, Barone G, Benati A, Beltramello A, Da Pian R: Treatment of cerebral arteriovenous malformations with a combination of preoperative embolization and surgery. Neurosurgery 1991;3:358–368.

44 Deruty R, Pelissou-Guyotat I, Mottolese C, Bascoulergue Y, Amat D: The combined management of cerebral arteriovenous malformations. Experience with 100 cases and review of the literature. Acta Neurochir (Wien) 1993;123:101–112.

45 Grzyska U, Westphal M, Zanella F: A joint protocol for the neurosurgical and neuroradiologic treatment of cerebral arteriovenous malformations: indications, technique and results in 76 cases. Surg Neurol 1993;40:476–484.

46 DeMerritt JS, Pile-Spellman J, Mast H: Outcome analysis of preoperative embolizations with N-butyl cyanoacrylate in cerebral arteriovenous malformations. AJNR Am J Neuroradiol 1995;16:1801–1807.

47 Fournier D, TerBrugge KG, Willinsky R, Lasjaunias P, Montanera W: Endovascular treatment of intracerebral arteriovenous malformations: experience in 49 cases. J Neurosurg 1995;75:228–233.

48 Debrun GM, Aletich V, Ausman JI, Charbel F, Dujovny M: Embolization of the nidus of brain arteriovenous malformations with n-butyl cyanoacrylate. Neurosurgery 1997;40:112–121.

49 Pelz DM, Fox AJ, Vinuela F, Drake CC, Ferguson GG: Preoperative embolization of brain AVMs with isobutyl-2 cyanoacrylate. AJNR Am J Neuroradiol 1988;9:757–764.

50 NBCA Trial Investigators: N-Butyl cyanoacrylate embolization of cerebral arteriovenous malformations: results of a prospective, randomized, multi-center trial. AJNR Am J Neuroradiol 2002;23:748–755.

51 Hurst RW, Berenstein A, Kupersmith MJ, Madrid M, Flamm ES: Deep central arteriovenous malformations of the brain: the role of endovascular treatment. J Neurosurg 1995;82:190–195.

52 Connors JJ, Wojak JC: Intracranial arteriovenous malformations: general considerations; in Connors JJ, Wojak JC (eds): Interventional Neuroradiology: Strategies and Practical Techniques. Philadelphia, Saunders, 1999, pp 227–240.

53 Gobin YP, Laurent A, Merienne L, Schlienger M, Aymard A, Houdart E, Casasco A, Lefkopoulos D, George B, Merland JJ: Treatment of brain arteriovenous malformations by embolization and radiosurgery. J Neurosurg 1996;85:19–28.
54 Valavanis A, Yasargil M: The endovascular treatment of brain arteriovenous malformations. Adv Tech Stand Neurosurg 1998;24:131–214.
55 Steinberg G, Fabrikant J, Marks M, Levy R, Frankel K, Phillips M, Shuer L, Silverberg G: Stereotactic heavy-charged-particle Bragg-peak radiation for intracranial arteriovenous malformations. N Engl J Med 1990;323:96–101.
56 Lunsford LD, Kondziolka D, Flickinger JC, Bissonette DJ, Jungreis CA, Maitz AH, Horton JA, Coffey RJ: Stereotactic radiosurgery for arteriovenous malformations of the brain. J Neurosurg 1991;75:512–524.
57 Colombo F, Pozza F, Chierego G, Casentini L, De Luca G, Francescon P: Linear accelerator radiosurgery of cerebral arteriovenous malformations: an update. Neurosurgery 1994;34:14–21.
58 Friedman WA, Bova FJ, Mendenhall WM: Linear accelerator radiosurgery for arteriovenous malformations: the relationship of size to outcome. J Neurosurg 1995;82:180–189.
59 Karlsson B, Lindquest C, Steiner L: Prediction of obliteration after gamma knife surgery for cerebral arteriovenous malformations. Neurosurgery 1997;40:425–431.
60 Pollock BE, Flickinger JC, Lunsford LD, Maitz AH, Kondziolka D: Factors associated with successful arteriovenous malformation radiosurgery. Neurosurgery 1998;42:1239–1244.
61 Schlienger M, Atlan D, Lefkopoulos D, Merienne L, Touboul E, Missir O, Nataf F, Mammar H, Platoni K, Grandjean P, Foulquier JN, Huart J, Oppenheim C, Meder JF, Houdart E, Merland JJ: Linac radiosurgery for cerebral arteriovenous malformations: results in 169 patients. Int J Radiat Oncol Biol Phys 2000;46:1135–1142.
62 Friedman WA, Bova FJ, Bollampally S, Bradshaw P: Analysis of factors predictive of success or complications in arteriovenous malformation radiosurgery. Neurosurgery 2003;52:296–307.
63 Mathis JA, Barr JD, Horton JA, Jungreis CA, Lunsford LD, Kondziolka DS, Vincent D, Pentheny S: The efficacy of particulate embolization combined with stereotactic radiosurgery for treatment of large arteriovenous malformations of the brain. Am J Neuroradiol 1995;16:299–306.
64 Steiner L, Lindquist C, Adler JR, Torner JC, Alves W, Steiner M: Clinical outcome of radiosurgery for cerebral arteriovenous malformations. J Neurosurg 1992;77:1–8.
65 Pollock BE, Kondziolka D, Lunsford LD, Bissonette DJ, Flickinger JC: Repeat stereotactic radiosurgery of arteriovenous malformations: factors associated with incomplete obliteration. Neurosurgery 1996;38:318–324.
66 Marks MP, Lane B, Steinberg GK, Fabrikant JI, Levy RP, Frankel KA, Phillips MH: Endovascular treatment of cerebral arteriovenous malformations following radiosurgery. AJNR Am J Neuroradiol 1993;14:197–303.
67 Steinberg GK, Chang SD, Levy RP, Marks MP, Frankel K, Marcellus M: Surgical resection of large incompletely treated intracranial arteriovenous malformations following stereotactic radiosurgery. J Neurosurg 1996;84:920–928.
68 Kusske JA, Kelly WA: Embolization and reduction of the 'steal' syndrome in cerebral arteriovenous malformations. J Neurosurg 1974;40:313–321.
69 Fox AJ, Girvin JP, Vinuela F, Drake CG: Rolandic arteriovenous malformations: improvement in limb function by IBC embolization. AJNR Am J Neuroradiol 1985;6:575–582.
70 Pollock BE, Flickinger JC, Lunsford LD, Bissonette DJ, Kondziolka D: Hemorrhage after stereotactic radiosurgery of cerebral arteriovenous malformations. Neurosurgery 1996;38: 659–661.
71 Han PP, Ponce FA, Spetzler RF: Intention-to-treat analysis of Spetzler-Martin grades IV and V arteriovenous malformations: natural history and treatment paradigm. J Neurosurg 2003;98:3–7.
72 Molyneux A, Kerr R, Stratton I, Sandercock P, Clarke M, Shrimpton J, Holman R, International Subarachnoid Aneurysm Trial (ISAT) Collaborative Group: International Subarachnoid Aneurysm Trial (ISAT) of neurosurgical clipping versus endovascular coiling in 2143 patients with ruptured intracranial aneurysms: a randomised trial. Lancet 2002;360:1267–1274.
73 Kassel NF, Torner JC, Jane JA, Haley ECJ, Adams HP: The international cooperative study on the timing of aneurysm surgery. 2. Surgical results. J Neurosurg 1990;73:37–47.

74 Johnston SC, Dudley RA, Gress DR, Ono L: Surgical and endovascular treatment of unruptured cerebral aneurysms at university hospitals. Neurology 1999;52:1799–1805.
75 Johnston SC, Wilson CV, Highashida RT, Dowd CF, McDermott MW, Applebury CB, Farley TL, Gress DR: Endovascular and surgical treatment of unruptured cerebral aneurysms: comparison of risks. Ann Neurol 2000;49:682–684.
76 Johnston SC, Zhao S, Dudley RA, Berman MF, Gress DR: Treatment of unruptured cerebral aneurysms in California. Stroke 2001;32:597–605.
77 Coward LF, Featherstone RL, Brown MM: Percutaneous transluminal angioplasty and stenting for carotid artery stenosis. Cochrane Database Syst Rev 2004;2:CD000515.
78 Brooks WH, McClure RR, Jones MR, Coleman TL, Breathitt L: Carotid angioplasty and stenting versus carotid endarterectomy for treatment of asymptomatic carotid stenosis: a randomized trial in a community hospital. Neurosurgery 2004;54:318–324.

Robert H. Rosenwasser, MD, FACS, Professor and Chairman
Department of Neurological Surgery
909 Walnut Street, Third Floor
Philadelphia, PA 19107 (USA)
Tel. +1 215 503 7004, Fax +1 215 503 7038, E-Mail Robert.Rosenwasser@mail.tju.edu

Pollock BE (ed): Guiding Neurosurgery by Evidence.
Prog Neurol Surg. Basel, Karger, 2006, vol 19, pp 123–134

Evidence-Based Guidelines in Lumbar Spine Surgery

Daniel K. Resnick[a], *Michael C. Groff*[b]

[a]Department of Neurological Surgery, University of Wisconsin, Madison, Wisc.,
[b]Department of Neurological Surgery, University of Indiana, Indianapolis, Ind., USA

Abstract

Lumbar fusion is a commonly performed procedure for the treatment of painful instability of the spine, usually manifest as chronic low back pain. The safety, efficacy, and cost of these procedures have been questioned in the professional and lay press. Recently, evidence based medicine techniques have been used to investigate the role of lumbar fusion for the treatment of a variety of spinal disorders. This chapter describes the general principles and procedures used for the development of evidence based guidelines for the performance of lumbar fusion.

The number of lumbar fusion procedures performed in the United States has increased substantially over the last several years and exhibited an upswing in the late 1990s [1]. There are distinct regional differences in the rate of fusions performed per 1,000 patients, a fact that has been interpreted in support of the hypothesis that fusion is overused. Recent editorials in the popular press [2] and general medical literature [1] have strongly condemned a perceived overutilization of lumbar fusion and have suggested that the increase in the frequency of fusion surgery noted over the last decade is a result of financial incentives to surgeons and instrumentation companies [2]. This condemnation is largely based on an apparent lack of evidence to support the role of fusion for the treatment of low back pain. Indeed, Gibson et al. [3] , in the 1999 Cochrane review stated: 'There is no scientific evidence on the effectiveness of any form of surgical decompression or fusion for degenerative lumbar spondylosis compared with natural history, placebo, or conservative management.' Third party payors, plaintiffs attorneys, journalists, and politicians have responded to such statements in a predictable fashion.

This chapter will focus on a review of the medical evidence available concerning the role of lumbar fusion for the treatment of chronic low back pain in patients without neurological deficit or significant spinal deformity. As such, the chapter is limited in scope. However, it is hoped that through this example the reader will be better able to understand the true strengths and limitations of evidence-based literature reviews as they apply to surgery of the lumbar spine.

Evidence-Based Medicine and the Low Back Pain Patient

The phrase 'evidence-based medicine' refers to the practice of medicine based upon the best available information in the literature. Evidence-based medicine does not refer to the 'ideal' or 'correct' practice of medicine. Literature cannot be interpreted in the absence of common sense and clinical experience. A frequently cited example of the inappropriate application of evidence-based medicine techniques is the assertion that there is no scientific evidence on the effectiveness of parachute use for life preservation following falls from aircraft [4]. Indeed, no randomized controlled trial or even a well-designed cohort comparison has ever been performed to provide such evidence. A less fanciful example of the limitations of literature-based guidelines concerns the evacuation of symptomatic intracranial epidural hematomas. The surgical head injury guidelines recommend removal of such hematomas at an option level [5] (supported only by low-quality or controversial evidence). This situation exists simply because no ethical surgeon would withhold available treatment from a patient with a symptomatic epidural hematoma, so no control group exists for comparison. Therefore, just because a treatment is not supported by high-quality medical evidence does not mean that a treatment has no value.

Other potential difficulties faced while trying to derive meaningful conclusions from the literature include the pace of technological development and the limitations imposed by the application of standardized outcome measures. Evolving technologies and techniques are, by definition, new and evolving. Therefore, the use of such techniques is not generally supported by high-quality medical evidence. When high-quality studies are available, they are almost always funded by the manufacturer of the device in question and run by investigators with a financial stake in the outcome of the study.

A number of commonly used, responsive, validated, and reliable outcome measures are available for the assessment of outcomes following lumbar fusion [6–19]. The use of such outcome measures allows for a comparison of different treatment strategies. Theoretically, if one treatment works better than another, then the outcomes achieved with the superior treatment should be measurably different from those achieved with the inferior treatment. Depending upon how the outcome measure is utilized, however, this may not always be the case. The limitations of commonly employed outcome measures may be illustrated by considering the advantages and disadvantages of minimally incisional technologies for the performance of lumbar fusion. It is a fairly standard practice for editorial boards to require a certain length of patient follow-up in clinical series. For example, the journal *Spine* generally requires a clinical manuscript to describe at least a 2-year follow-up following fusion procedures in order to be considered for publication. If a functional outcome measure is applied to patients who have undergone fusion procedures two or more years following surgery, any potential short-term benefit related to a minimally incisional approach would not be detected. Therefore, the potential advantages of a minimally incisional approach (shorter hospital stay, less acute pain) would not be reflected as an improvement in functional outcome (see fig. 1).

Similarly, lumbar fusion surgery is not performed on patients with normal lumbar spinal anatomy. In order for a fusion procedure to be contemplated, some evidence of abnormality, usually a form of instability must be demonstrated. Patients with instability of the spine are different from their peers in that they have 'bad backs'. Surgical treatment directed at a single level may well provide temporary amelioration of symptoms, however over time the strength of this beneficial effect may deteriorate due to the natural history of degenerative spine disease. Therefore a beneficial effect noted 1, 2 or 5 years following surgery may not be present 10 years following surgery. In this case, an outcome study performed 10 years following fusion surgery would fail to demonstrate that surgery had a beneficial effect (fig. 1). Does this truly mean that the patients did not benefit from the procedure? Additionally, outcome measures appropriate for one population undergoing lumbar fusion may not be appropriate for other populations undergoing fusion. For example, return to work rate may be a valid, reliable, and responsive outcome measure for patients undergoing anterior lumbar interbody fusion. Is this outcome measure appropriate when we are studying the results of fusion versus no fusion in patients undergoing decompression for lumbar stenosis?

Another significant limitation encountered in the interpretation of the medical literature relates to the definition of a clinically relevant outcome measure. For example, in a study of the use of bone morphogenetic proteins (BMP) as a substitute for autograft, the authors note a 'significant' decrease in blood loss in the BMP group [20–22]. The magnitude of this decrease was

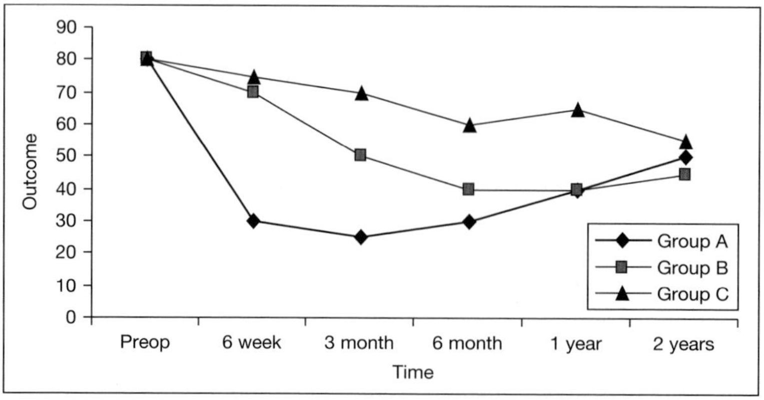

Fig. 1. Outcome measures over time. This graph depicts the clinical response of a hypothetical population of patients with low back pain divided into three treatment groups and followed for 2 years. Patients in group A were treated with intensive physiotherapy, counseling, weight loss and smoking cessation. This group of patients had a very slow resolution of back pain over a number of years. Patients in group B were treated with a noninstrumented PLF. They took some time to get over the operation, but noted a significant improvement (compared to group A) at 6 months and 1 year following surgery. Their improvement leveled out however, and at the 2-year mark their functional outcome was similar to group A. Patients in group C underwent a minimally invasive interbody fusion with percutaneous fixation. They recovered from the surgery very quickly and enjoyed significant resolution of their pain very soon after surgery. The improvement was static, however, and over time their functional outcome reverted towards the other groups due to the natural history of degenerative disc disease (progressive degeneration). Does the faster resolution of pain enjoyed by group C warrant the costs of the procedure? Does the fact that the results are similar at 2 years mean that there is no value associated with the decrease in pain and improved function in the intervening years? See text for more discussion.

66 ml per patient. Is this a clinically relevant benefit? Does this justify an extra USD 5,000 per patient? Conversely, Fritzell et al. [23], in a randomized series comparing fusion techniques for low back pain, found that there was significant functional improvement in 70% of patients treated with posterolateral fusion (PLF) with pedicle screws compared to 60% of those patients treated with PLF alone. The paper was substantially underpowered to detect this level of improvement (see below), and therefore this difference in outcomes was not found to be significant. Is this degree of improvement worthwhile? If so, what does it mean if an underpowered trial failed to demonstrate a significant effect?

Despite these limitations of evidence-based literature review, it is imperative that we examine the literature to establish clinical guidelines. These reviews provide snapshots of the state of the literature regarding a particular topic. The guidelines produced are reflections of the peer-reviewed literature and provide valuable guidance regarding what is truly known on a particular treatment or diagnostic test. They serve to improve the literature itself through critique and grading of individual papers and through the suggestion of future research directions designed to fill noticeable gaps in our collective knowledge base. These techniques are also being used by agencies outside of medicine to determine which procedures are paid for, which procedures are within the 'standard of care', and which devices are approved for use. If we physicians are not intimately familiar with the strengths, weaknesses, and conclusions reached in our own literature, we will forfeit our ability to participate in the formulation of health care policy.

Is Lumbar Fusion an Effective Treatment for Low Back Pain?

There are multiple indications for fusion, multiple techniques for the achievement of fusion, a variety of diagnostic tests to determine eligibility for fusion procedures, and numerous methods of assessing outcome. The literature concerning lumbar fusion has generally been regarded as a morass of low-quality heterogeneous reports describing different procedures performed on different patient populations. Some authors have concluded that there is, in fact, no evidence to support the use of fusion as a treatment for painful degenerative disease of the spine [3]. In January 2003, the AANS/CNS Joint Section on Disorders of the Spine and Peripheral Nerves was charged by the leadership of the CNS to develop evidence-based guidelines for the performance of lumbar fusion. The section responded by funding a guideline effort utilizing similar methodology to the cervical spine injury guidelines published in March 2002 [24]. These guidelines were produced through a collaborative effort between the spine section and the North American Spine Society and are scheduled for publication in the near future. These guidelines consist of 17 separate papers dealing with specific aspects of lumbar fusion for degenerative disease. Although a full discussion of the guidelines is beyond the scope of this chapter, the process will be illustrated through a consideration of the surgical management of low back pain.

The strongest medical evidence, here labeled as 'class I medical evidence', in support for a given treatment is derived from well-designed and appropriately powered randomized controlled clinical trials. If a randomized controlled clinical trial is poorly designed or underpowered, the quality of the evidence that it provides is downgraded to class II or class III medical evidence. When trials of similar quality provide conflicting conclusions, the design of the study is examined closely in order to determine which study is better designed. The COHORT group has published a set of criteria for the grading of clinical trials [25] which allows for a rational application of this principle.

There have been two randomized controlled clinical trials published that describe a comparison between the efficacy of surgery (fusion) and nonsurgical management of chronic low back pain due to degenerative disease of the lumbar spine at L4–L5, L5–S1, or both levels. Fritzell et al. [26] published the results of a multicenter randomized controlled trial from the Swedish Lumbar Spine Study Group in 2001. These authors assumed that very few patients would improve with conservative care and that a modest proportion of patients treated surgically would improve. They performed a power analysis based upon this premise in order to have an 80% power to detect a significant difference in the effect of surgery versus the effect of nonsurgical treatment (in other words, they determined how much of an improvement they thought would be clinically relevant, and figured out how many patients they needed to include in order to be able to detect that degree of improvement 80% of the time). In this study, 294 patients with disabling back pain who were felt to be surgical candidates were randomized to conservative care (physical therapy supplemented with education and other pain-relieving technologies at the discretion of the treating physician), or one of three surgical treatment arms. Patients were required to have suffered from back pain for at least 2 years and to have radiographic and clinical evidence of spondylosis at L4–5, L5–S1, or both levels. The groups were comparable in all demographic variables measured with the exception of a higher incidence of medical comorbidity in the surgical group. Patients were followed for 2 years with intermediate evaluations at 6 months and at 1 year following onset of treatment. Outcomes were assessed using multiple well-validated outcome measures including pain visual analogue scales, the Oswestry Low Back Pain Questionnaire, the Million Visual Analogue Scale, the General Function Scale (GFS), Work Status, a patient satisfaction survey, and an independent functional assessment by a second spinal surgeon [26].

Follow-up was achieved in 98% of patients. Appropriate statistical analysis was performed based upon the type of data derived from the different outcome measures. The surgical group did significantly better in terms of pain relief, degree of disability as measured by the Oswestry, Million, and GFS, return to work status, and degree of satisfaction reported by the patients and by the independent observer. Statistical analysis was rigorous, employing 'intention to treat' as well as a 'worst case' scenarios. In short, all primary outcome measures evaluated in the study were significantly improved in the surgical group compared to the nonsurgical group [26]. This study is therefore felt to provide class I evidence demonstrating that lumbar fusion is associated with better outcomes than standard conservative care for appropriately selected patients.

The study of Fritzell et al. [26] was criticized by proponents of various nonsurgical therapies. For example, Mooney [27] commented that the study was unfairly biased against conservative care because the patients had already failed a trial of the same type of therapy prior to entry in the study. This criticism appears to be valid, given the a priori assumptions made by the Fritzell group in their initial power analysis. This criticism does not, however, diminish the finding that patients treated with lumbar fusion have superior clinical outcomes compared to similar patients treated with usual medical care or those left to suffer the natural history of disabling low back pain.

In 2003, Brox et al. [28] conducted a smaller (i.e. less powerful) randomized study evaluating the relative efficacy of instrumented PLF versus a specific protocol of cognitive intervention and physical therapy. The primary outcome measure used was a modified Oswestry Disability Index (modified for the Norwegian population) [29]. Secondary outcome measures included pain visual analogue scales, daily use of medication, GFS, Waddel's Fear Avoidance Belief Questionnaire, and a patient satisfaction score. Outcomes were assessed by physical therapists or rehabilitation physicians at 1 year following initiation of treatment.

Patients enrolled in the surgical arm were treated with instrumented PLF. The patients enrolled in the physiotherapy arm underwent a program specifically designed for patients with low back pain that was felt to be more effective than standard conservative care based on a pilot study performed by the authors [30]. This program included significant cognitive therapy designed to lower patient fear as well as supervised physiotherapy averaging 25 h per week for 8 weeks. Because of the intensity of the program, most patients stayed at the treatment center in patient hotels. This intensive course was followed by a home program based on the exercises prescribed in the supervised portion. In addition, patients in the physiotherapy group were offered individual consultations, lessons, group therapy sessions, and participation in peer-led discussion groups.

Sixty-four patients were randomized, 37 to surgery and 27 to physiotherapy. There were more men randomized to the surgical group, otherwise the groups were comparable. The 1-year follow-up rate was 97%. Both groups improved significantly from baseline on all outcome measures. The improvement in the primary outcome measure, the modified ODI, in the surgical group was 15.6 and the improvement in the physiotherapy group was 13.3. There were very large confidence intervals noted in this as well as other outcome measures assessed. The difference in the degree of improvement between the surgical and physiotherapy group was not found to be significant. The surgical group did do significantly better in terms of relief of lower limb pain and tended to do better than the physiotherapy group in terms of improvement in back pain, emotional distress, and overall success ratings by both the patient and the independent observer. The physiotherapy group scored better fear avoidance activity and work as well as in fingertip-floor distance. Nonsignificant trends were also seen in favor of the physiotherapy group in terms of the GFS and life satisfaction score [28].

The authors interpret their findings as demonstrating an equivalence between their program of physiotherapy and lumbar fusion. Given the small size of the study groups and the very large confidence intervals reported in the paper, the evidence provided by the paper is considered to provide class III evidence concerning the relative efficacy of fusion versus intensive physiotherapy. The paper does not address the utility of fusion as a means to alter the natural history of low back pain and is significantly underpowered to detect any differences between any treatments that are even remotely similar (see below). The relevance of the paper may be further questioned given the intensity of the treatment used in the physiotherapy group. It is doubtful that such a program is available to the vast majority of patients treated for low back pain.

Sample Size, Clinically Relevant Effect, and Pedicle Screws

The importance of sample size and the definition of 'clinically relevant effect' cannot be overstated. A large randomized controlled clinical study may demonstrate a 'statistically significant effect' of a treatment modality. If the sample size is large enough, a small difference in outcomes may reach significance (see fig. 2). Consider the NASCIS spinal cord injury studies [31–35]. In these studies, large numbers of patients were enrolled and a beneficial effect of methylprednisolone on clinical outcome measured with the ASIA scale was identified (in a subgroup of patients). The magnitude of the improvement was small, however, and the use of methylprednisolone was associated with an increased risk of complications [31–35]. Is the small potential benefit of methylprednisolone use worth the increased risk of complications? Not all clinicians believe so [36–38]. Here is where the clinician must make a judgement as to the clinical importance of a 4-point improvement in the ASIA scale versus an increased risk of sepsis. Conversely, a substantial beneficial effect may not be recognized if sample sizes are too small (fig. 2).

Previously, we discussed the study by Fritzell et al. [26] which examined the role of lumbar fusion. These authors performed a power analysis to determine how many patients they would need to include in their study in order to have a reasonable chance of detecting a significant effect. They assumed that the control patients would do very poorly and that the treated patients would do moderately well. They made several assumptions as to what degree of Oswestry or GFS improvement would be considered relevant and were able to demonstrate a significant effect between the surgical and nonsurgical arms [26]. These same authors then

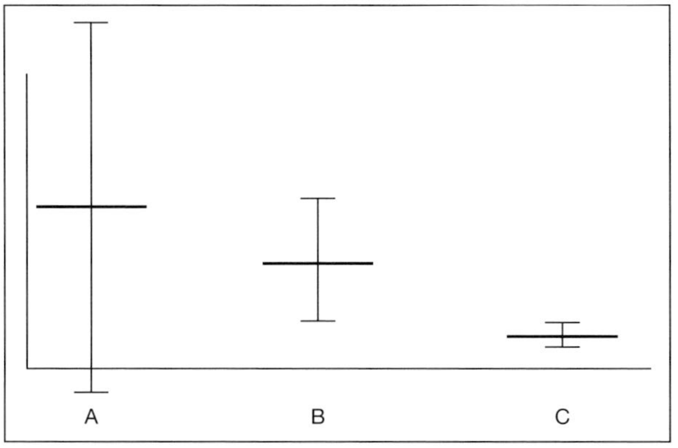

Fig. 2. The deception of power. This graph, adapted from Matthews and Farewell [39], illustrates the problems encountered when trying to interpret studies which are either underpowered or overpowered. On this arbitrary scale, a higher value is associated with a greater beneficial effect. Assume that the heavy line represents the true effect of a treatment. Treatment A was studied in a small randomized controlled trial and initially appeared to be very beneficial. Unfortunately, because of a relatively small sample size, there was a large variance within the sample tested. Because of this, a relatively large treatment effect was found to be nonsignificant. Treatment C was studied in a large multicenter study. Because of the large number of patients involved, a very small treatment effect was found to be significant. Therefore, in this example, treatment C would be considered more efficacious than treatment A despite the fact that the absolute degree of improvement seen in treatment C was less than that seen in treatment A. Treatment B was found to have a moderate effect and was detected as significant when studied in an appropriately powered clinical trial.

published an analysis of their results within the surgical groups. They compared a noninstrumented PLF group to a PLF group supplemented with pedicle screws and to a circumferential fusion group. They found that there were no significant differences between the groups in terms of functional outcomes and that complication rates were higher in the instrumented and circumferential groups [23].

When one examines the results presented in the Fritzell paper, however, it becomes apparent that the group of patients treated with pedicle screw fixation did score better than the PLF alone group on most of the outcome measures reported, including the Oswestry, GFS, and patient satisfaction surveys. There was a relative 40% increase in the degree of improvement on the Oswestry in the group treated with pedicle screw fixation and an increase in successful outcomes from 60 to 70% (PLF alone vs. PLF plus pedicle screws). Is a 40% increase in the degree of improvement on the Oswestry scale or a 16% improvement in rate of good outcomes clinically relevant? If so, why was this difference in outcome not detected as significant?

The problem here is that the Fritzell study was designed to detect a difference between a group of patients who enjoyed a moderate improvement and a group of patients who did not improve much at all. While the authors were able to detect just such a difference between the surgical and nonsurgical arms, the study was underpowered to detect differences between a group of patients who enjoyed a moderate improvement and a group of patients who had a better improvement. A power analysis reveals that in order to have an reasonable chance (80%) of detecting a statistically significant difference between a group of patients who achieve a good outcome 60% of the time and another group of patients who achieve a good outcome 70% of the time, over 350 patients are required in each group (http://calculators.stat.ucla.edu/powercalc). Playing with the numbers, it is possible to calculate that the Fritzell study had only a 42% chance of detecting an effect of this magnitude. Therefore, should we interpret the negative results in the Fritzell study as definitive evidence that the addition of pedicle screws does not improve outcome? The answer is no. The absence of a positive effect in an underpowered study cannot be interpreted as anything except circumstantial evidence (class III) regarding the lack of a treatment effect.

There are multiple examples of these types of design flaws in the literature concerning lumbar fusion. Unfortunately for the spine surgeon and the patient with low back pain, these design flaws create the impression that many of the procedures we do are not effective. Third party payors, politicians, and our patients are demanding justification for the potentially risky and certainly expensive procedures that we are performing on otherwise healthy individuals. There are really no ethical issues preventing the performance of appropriately designed randomized controlled studies to examine the relative efficacy of various fusion procedures to noninstrumented PLF in the many subpopulations of patients undergoing fusion for low back pain. The challenge is to determine the right procedure for a given patient population, define a clinically relevant difference in outcome using reliable and valid outcome measures, design a study with adequate power, and perform the study in an era of burdensome HIPAA regulations and public scrutiny.

Improving the Literature

In order to improve our literature, we must design studies that are geared towards answering reasonable questions. We need to study techniques in specific patient populations and compare these techniques to 'gold standard' techniques or to the natural history of the disease process. For example, the use of interbody techniques as a treatment for low back pain is probably not best studied in the elderly patient with stenosis and degenerative spondylolisthesis. Conversely, noninstrumented PLF has been found to be an effective treatment for low back pain and may be an appropriate control group for studies looking at interbody techniques in the younger low back pain population. Clinical insight combined with expertise in clinical trial design will be required in order to provide high-quality medical evidence to support the procedures we perform to improve the quality of life for our patients.

References

1 Deyo RA, Nachemson A, Mirza SK: Spinal-fusion surgery – the case for restraint. N Engl J Med 2004;350:722–726.

2 Abelson R, Peterson M: An operation to ease back pain bolsters the bottom line, too. New York Times, Dec 31, 2003.

3 Gibson JN, Grant IC, Waddell G: The Cochrane review of surgery for lumbar disc prolapse and degenerative lumbar spondylosis. Spine 1999;24:1820–1832.

4 Smith GCS, Pell JP: Parachute use to prevent death and major trauma related to gravitational challenge: systematic review of randomised controlled trials. BMJ 2003;327:1459–1461.

5 Bullock MR, Chestnut R, Ghajar J, Gordon D, Hartl R, Newell DW, Servadei F, Walters BC, Wilberger JE: Surgical Management of Acute Epidural Hematoma. Neurosurgery 2006;58(suppl 2):7–15.

6 Deyo RA: Comparative validity of the sickness impact profile and shorter scales for functional assessment in low back pain. Spine 1986;11:951–954.

7 Deyo RA, Andersson G, Bombardier C, Cherkin DC, Keller RB, Lee CK, Liang MH, Lipscomb B, Shekelle P, Spratt KF, et al: Outcome measures for studying patients with low back pain. Spine 1994;19(18 suppl):2032S–2036S.

8 Fairbank JC, Couper J, Davies JB, O'Brien JP: The Oswestry low back pain disability questionnaire. Physiotherapy 1980;66:271–273.

9 Harper AC, Harper DA, Lambert LJ, de Klerk NH, Andrews HB, Ross FM, Straker LJ, Lo SK: Development and validation of the Curtin Back Screening Questionnaire (CBSQ): a discriminative disability measure. Pain 1995;60:73–81.

10 Lawlis GF, Cuencas R, Selby D, McCoy CE: The development of the Dallas Pain Questionnaire: an assessment of the impact of spinal pain on behavior. Spine 1989;14:511–516.

11 Leclaire R, Blier F, Fortin L, Proulx R: A cross-sectional study comparing the Oswestry and Roland-Morris Functional Disability scales in two populations of patients with low back pain of different levels of severity. Spine 1997;22:68–71.

12 Manniche C, Asmussen K, Lauritsen B, Vinterberg H, Kreiner S, Jordan A: Low back pain rating scale: validation of a tool for assessment of low back pain. Pain 1994;57:317–326.

13 Million R, Hall W, Nilsen KH, Baker RD, Jayson MI: Assessment of the progress of the back-pain patient. Spine 1982;7:204–208.

14 Roland M, Morris R: A study of the natural history of back pain. I. Development of a reliable and sensitive measure of disability in low-back pain. Spine 1983;8:141–144.

15 Ruta DA, Garratt A, Wardlaw D, Russell IT: Developing a valid and reliable measure of health outcome for patients with low back pain. Spine 1994;19:1887–1896.

16 Salen BA, Spangfort E, Nygren AL, Nordemar R: The Disability Rating Index: an instrument for the assessment of disability in clinical settings. J Clin Epidemiol 1994;47:1423–1435.

17 Stucki G, Daltroy L, Liang MH, Lipson SJ, Fossel AH, Katz JN: Measurement properties of a self-administered outcome measure in lumbar spinal stenosis. Spine 1996;21:796–803.

18 Waddell G, Main CJ: Assessment of severity in low-back disorders. Spine 1984;9:204–208.

19 Ware J Jr, Kosinski M, Keller SD: A 12-item short-form health survey: construction of scales and preliminary tests of reliability and validity. Med Care 1996;34:220–233.

20 Burkus JK, Heim SE, Gornet MF, Zdeblick TA: Is INFUSE bone graft superior to autograft bone? An integrated analysis of clinical trials using the LT-CAGE lumbar tapered fusion device. J Spinal Disord Tech 2003;16:113–122.

21 Burkus JK, Transfeldt EE, Kitchel SH, Watkins RG, Balderston RA: Clinical and radiographic outcomes of anterior lumbar interbody fusion using recombinant human bone morphogenetic protein-2. Spine 2002;27:2396–2408.
22 Burkus JK, Dorchak JD, Sanders DL: Radiographic assessment of interbody fusion using recombinant human bone morphogenetic protein type 2. Spine 2003;28:372–377.
23 Fritzell P, Hagg O, Wessberg P, Nordwall A, Swedish Lumbar Spine Study Group: Chronic low back pain and fusion: a comparison of three surgical techniques: a prospective multicenter randomized study from the Swedish lumbar spine study group. Spine 2002;27:1131–1141.
24 Hadley MN, Walters BC, Grabb PA, Oyesiku NM, Przybylski GJ, Resnick DK, Ryken TC: Guidelines for the management of acute cervical spine and spinal cord injuries. Neurosurgery 2002;50(suppl):S2–S6.
25 Moher D, Schulz KF, Altman DG: The CONSORT statement: revised recommendations for improving the quality of reports of parallel-group randomised trials. Lancet 2001;357:1192–1194.
26 Fritzell P, Hagg O, Wessberg P, Nordwall A, Swedish Lumbar Spine Study Group: Lumbar fusion versus nonsurgical treatment for chronic low back pain: a multicenter randomized controlled trial from the Swedish Lumbar Spine Study Group. Spine 2001;26:2521.
27 Mooney V: Point of view. Spine 2001;26:2532–2533.
28 Brox IJ, Sorensen R, Friis A, Nygaard O, Indahl A, Keller A, Ingebrigtsen T, Eriksen HR, Holm I, Koller AK, Riise R, Reikeras O: Randomized clinical trial of lumbar instrumented fusion and cognitive intervention and exercises in patients with chronic low back pain and disc degeneration. Spine 2003;28:1913–1921.
29 Holm I, Friis A, Storheim K: Measuring self reported functional status and pain in patients with chronic low back pain by postal questionnaires: a reliability study. Spine 2003;28:828–833.
30 Brox IJ, Friis A, Holm I: Patients with chronic degenerative spinal disease: can conservative treatment reduce the waiting list for surgery? Tidsskr Nor Laegeforen 1999;119:1784–1787.
31 Bracken MB, Shepard MJ, Collins WF, et al: A randomized, controlled trial of methylprednisolone or naloxone in the treatment of acute spinal-cord injury. Results of the Second National Acute Spinal Cord Injury Study. N Engl J Med 1990;322:1405–1411.
32 Bracken MB, Shepard MJ, Collins WF Jr, Holford TR, Baskin DS, Eisenberg HM, et al: Methylprednisolone or naloxone treatment after acute spinal cord injury: 1-year follow-up data. Results of the second National Acute Spinal Cord Injury Study. J Neurosurg 1992;76:23–31.
33 Bracken MB, Shepard MJ, Holford TR, et al: Administration of methylprednisolone for 24 or 48 hours or tirilazad mesylate for 48 hours in the treatment of acute spinal cord injury. Results of the Third National Acute Spinal Cord Injury Randomized Controlled Trial. National Acute Spinal Cord Injury Study. JAMA 1997;277:1597–1604.
34 Bracken MB, Shepard MJ, Holford TR, et al: Methylprednisolone or tirilazad mesylate administration after acute spinal cord injury: 1-year follow-up. Results of the third National Acute Spinal Cord Injury randomized controlled trial. J Neurosurg 1998;89:699–706.
35 Bracken MB, Holford TR: Neurological and functional status 1 year after acute spinal cord injury: estimates of functional recovery in National Acute Spinal Cord Injury Study II from results modeled in National Acute Spinal Cord Injury Study III. J Neurosurg 2002;96(3 suppl):259–266.
36 Hurlbert RJ: Methylprednisolone for acute spinal cord injury: an inappropriate standard of care. J Neurosurg 2000;93(1 suppl):1–7.
37 Hurlbert RJ: The role of steroids in acute spinal cord injury: an evidence-based analysis. Spine 2001;26(24 suppl):S39–46.
38 Hurlbert RJ, Moulton R: Why do you prescribe methylprednisolone for acute spinal cord injury? A Canadian perspective and a position statement. Can J Neurol Sci 2002;29:236–239.
39 Matthews DE, Farewell VT: Using and Understanding Medical Statistics, ed 3. Basel, Karger, 1996.

Daniel K. Resnick, MD
K4/834 Clinical Science Center
600 Highland Avenue
Madison, WI 53792 (USA)
Tel. +1 608 263 9651, Fax +1 608 263 1728, E-Mail Resnick@neurosurg.wisc.edu

Pollock BE (ed): Guiding Neurosurgery by Evidence.
Prog Neurol Surg. Basel, Karger, 2006, vol 19, pp 135–151

Spine: Minimally Invasive Techniques

Peter C. Gerszten, William C. Welch

Department of Neurological Surgery, University of Pittsburgh School of Medicine, UPMC Health System, Pittsburgh, Pa., USA

Abstract

Minimally invasive spine surgery decompression, arthrodesis, and instrumentation techniques are now being applied in a wide variety of percutaneous, laparoscopic and minimal access procedures. There is currently little longitudinal long-term data on these procedures to document their efficacy, indications, limitations or complications as compared to standard open techniques. Further complicating such direct comparisons is that widely used spine outcomes instruments often do not capture the relative benefits of these new procedures. It is only through randomized trials that the potential benefits of these procedures be substantiated in order to justify the sometimes significant increased costs associated with them.

There has been a gradual development over time of minimally invasive surgical techniques applied to the field of spine surgery [1]. Such techniques follow a natural trend in surgery to minimize the injury to normal tissue while obtaining the same or a better surgical outcome. The new wave in recent years of minimally invasive spinal procedures is not a revolution, but rather an evolution of familiar, time-proven operative techniques [2]. Such an attitude towards these new techniques helps to understand the relative paucity of rigorous evidence-based outcomes assessments of these techniques prior to their widespread adoption.

By marrying modern medical technology to traditional spinal approaches, the classical goals of open spinal surgery can now be effectively and reproducibly accomplished through much smaller corridors and with far less iatrogenic damage to the vital dorsal musculoligamentous complex [2]. Innovation in surgical treatment reflects either the application of existing knowledge, techniques, or technology in new ways or the acquisition and application of new knowledge to fundamentally redefine the management of a condition [3]. Both types of innovations will be reviewed in this chapter. For example, the use of the endoscope in spinal procedures is based upon its prior success in surgery elsewhere in the body and is an example of the former type of innovation. On the other hand, the techniques of vertebroplasty and kyphoplasty represent the latter form of innovation.

There is still some debate over the definition of 'minimally invasive spine surgery'. Indeed, Fessler [4] points out that many of these procedures being developed do not rely on new and untested technologies to achieve their surgical results. For example, after the target has been reached, procedures such as microendoscopic discectomy involve the use of standard surgical instruments and techniques. In this respect, the crucial aspect of the surgical procedure is not minimal at all; it is exactly the same as the equivalent open procedure. However, 'minimal access' techniques have been used to access the surgical target. Therefore, 'minimal access spine surgery' is probably a more accurate term to describe this family of procedures [4].

Not only is there some debate over the term 'minimally invasive', there is also disagreement regarding the definition of what actually constitutes 'surgery'. Many of these minimally invasive techniques, especially those that are percutaneous such as vertebroplasty and intradiscal electrothermal therapy (IDET), are more commonly performed by interventional radiologists and anesthesiologists than they are by spine orthopedic and neurosurgeons. The procedures included in this chapter are those that are considered to be commonly performed by surgeons who operate on the spine.

Outcome Evaluation of Minimally Invasive Techniques

Outcome Comparison

Well-established reliable and validated outcome instruments and techniques already exist for the proper evidence-based evaluation of most surgical spinal techniques [5, 6]. In contrast, most evaluations of minimally invasive spinal surgery techniques have focused on variables such as decreases in operating times, blood loss, postoperative pain, medication use, length of hospital stays, and costs (see table 1) [4]. The improved 'quality' of these surgical techniques can be measured in many ways, including decreased risk related to the procedure, more reliable and/or easier achievement of the surgical objective, superior short-term and/or more durable long-term outcomes, less pain and quicker recovery, and more efficient achievement of the surgical objective, with respect to the resources consumed [3]. However, standard disease-specific

Table 1. Common outcome measures for minimally invasive spine techniques

Postoperative incisional pain
Pain scores
Size of incision
Length of hospital stay
Blood loss
Patient satisfaction scores
Patients' willingness to repeat surgery under similar circumstances
Postoperative analgesic use
Operative times
Time until return to unrestricted full activity
Cost
Similar long-term results compared to conventional techniques

spinal outcome instruments such as the Oswestry Low Back Pain Disability Questionnaire, North American Spine Society Questionnaire as well as others from the Compendium of Outcome Instruments for Assessment and Research of Spinal Disorders of the North American Spine Society [7, 8] are simply neither sensitive nor specific enough to measure such marginal improvements in patient outcomes. In other words, they were not designed to measure (and thus compare) such outcomes as length of stay in the hospital, extent of postoperative pain, amount of postoperative analgesic use, or time until return to normal activities. It must be understood that the development of these new techniques is not necessarily being driven by a problem with the current standard surgical technique. Therefore, one would not necessarily expect that commonly used patient-reported outcome questionnaires would show a statistically significant improvement over standard techniques. This becomes problematic even for rather straightforward assessments such as hospital length of stay. For procedures such as traditional open microdiscectomies using loupe or microscopic magnification, which are routinely performed in an outpatient setting with minimal blood loss, a comparison to endoscopic microdiscectomy examining these two variables would not show any benefit.

Proper outcomes assessment of these minimally invasive spine techniques is further complicated by the difficulty of *timing* of patient evaluation. Outcome instruments such as visual analog scales for pain only represent a single time point. If a particular minimally invasive spine procedure improves pain in the immediate postoperative procedure, a visual analog scale data point acquired during the first postoperative visit at 3 weeks would simply not capture that improvement. What might have been a significant improvement for the patient regarding their quality of life in the immediate postoperative period would not have been captured during a standard outcomes assessment of the technique. Therefore, not only might the instruments not be sensitive to relative improvements in patient outcomes, great attention must be placed upon when in the perioperative period outcome data were collected from the patient.

One final issue that makes an evidence-based evaluation difficult for these techniques is that there is often no gold standard medical or surgical treatment for many of these disease processes. Class I outcome data for the traditional surgical approach to many of these disorders is lacking [9]. In addition, there is already a tremendous variation in the technique used by surgeons for even the most common of spinal surgical procedures such as the microdiscectomy. Such a wide variation in technique precludes the evaluation of large numbers of patients treated by different surgeons, even at the same institution, in any given published series. Most published data on these minimally invasive techniques represent class 5 case series technical reports that focus on a description of methodology and complication avoidance rather than quality outcomes assessment [9]. The benefits to the patients are usually *implied* to the reader as an obvious result of the perceived improvement in technique.

Cost Comparisons

Cost evaluations for these minimally invasive spine techniques are incredibly complex and difficult to analyze. It is very difficult to accurately calculate the financial benefits, if any, of these procedures. There is sometimes a shift in cost back to the hospital such as longer operating times or capital equipment purchases that are often not considered in the published reports of these techniques. One must take into account both direct as well as indirect costs when evaluating cost effectiveness. Proper cost-effective analyses require the acquisition of preference-based measurements such as quality-adjusted life years [5]. Preference-based measurements such as standard gamble and time trade-off scaling methods are rarely obtained when evaluating minimally invasive spine techniques. Other quality of life outcome instrument simply do not allow for cost:benefit and cost-effectiveness analyses.

Aside from direct financial costs, many of these techniques require extensive investments of time and effort on the part of the surgeons in gaining the required technical skills (usually in animal or cadaver laboratory setting), and negotiating a substantial clinical experience ‘learning curve’. Such important variables and ‘costs’ (in terms of acquisition of appropriate skills and equipment) are almost impossible to capture when comparing these new techniques to more standard open ones.

Efficacy and Effectiveness

It cannot be validly concluded that the results reported in the literature by an expert in one of these techniques, even using the most rigorous standards, are generalizable for the average practitioner. These published results simply represent the unique experience of the authors, with their selection processes, their skills, their judgment, and their assessments [3]. This is the difference between *efficacy* and *effectiveness*. Efficacy reflects the level of benefit expected when health care services are applied under 'ideal' conditions of use. In contrast, effectiveness concerns the level of benefit when services are rendered under ordinary circumstances by average practitioners for typical patients [10]. Efficacy indicates the outcomes that can ultimately be achieved with a given health care service, and effectiveness reveals the outcomes that are presently reached. In other words, the patient outcomes demonstrated by a very experienced surgeon might not translate well in the hands of a less experienced surgeon. Complication rates might also be much higher. Furthermore, these same 'experts' who have developed and mastered these new techniques would be the least willing to perform a quality comparative outcome evaluation to more standard open techniques that would require their patients to agree to a randomization procedure.

Furthermore, there will always be a tendency toward bias in the reported literature on such techniques. The concept of 'bias' is especially important in an evidence-based evaluation of minimally invasive spine surgery for several unique reasons [11]. There is a clear 'selection bias' with respect to the selection of manuscripts addressing these 'hot topics' to be published in the neurosurgical and spine literature. There is also a 'selection bias' in the selection of the 'best' patients to be included in a study. Given that such technologies are often industry developed, there is also a 'commercial bias', including the intended or unintended inclusion or exclusion of data, manuscripts, or concepts on the basis of monetary or financial interest. The companies that develop these advanced technologies are more often interested in safety concerns than patient outcomes. They often rely more upon perceived benefits targeted at surgeons that will allow them to successfully market their product. Finally, there is significant 'personal bias' involved in the publication of the results of these new techniques that can intentionally or inadvertently lead to personal gain or self-aggrandizement and that can thus adversely influence the scientific literature [11].

One final problem that adds to the complexity for the proper evidence-based evaluation of these techniques must be mentioned. The 'current' use of any of these techniques represents a 'moving target'. The technology often is evolving so quickly that by the time a series of patients is published by a leading authority in the field, that authority has often gone on to use the next generation of technology available. Therefore, by the time an article is published and distributed, the methodologies described might no longer be the 'state-of-the-art' or even available for more widespread use. Patient selection criteria might also have changed. Patients' outcomes might correspondingly not be the same as well. This is a problem that is common among the surgical subspecialties applying minimally invasive technology to their field.

Selected Minimally Invasive Spinal Procedures

Any division of minimally invasive surgery of the spine is somewhat arbitrary and by nature cannot be all-inclusive. This chapter will try to evaluate some of the more commonly used techniques that have been evaluated in the peer-reviewed literature. As previously discussed, given the incredible variation in the ways in which these techniques are performed, dogmatic statements either supporting or refuting their benefits are impossible to make. Class I or class II evidence is currently lacking for many of these procedures [9]. The evolution and advancements in minimally invasive spinal surgery over the last 15 years has essentially mirrored that of traditional open procedures during the last century. Fundamental to the growth of posterior minimally invasive spinal techniques is the attempt to minimize iatrogenic injury associated with standard spinal open exposures.

Posterior Cervical Procedures

The effectiveness of posterior cervical laminoforaminotomy for decompression for the lateral recess and neural foramen has been well documented [12–14]. The use of a microendoscopic system for posterior cervical laminoforaminotomy was developed to overcome the limitations of the open procedure, namely a limited surgical view, difficulty in resecting uncovertebral osteophytes, limited visualization of the distal foramen, and often generous epidural venous bleeding [2]. Several class III and class IV studies have been published. Adamson [15] described his technique in 100 cases. He reported a 97% excellent or good result. Khoo and Gravori [2] reported a class III prospective nonrandomized comparison in 60 patients with open versus tubular endoscopic foraminotomies after a mean follow-up of 4.6 months. Both studies found shortened postoperative length of stays, decreased blood loss, minimal postoperative narcotic pain requirements, and a quicker return to unrestricted full activity in the endoscopic patient group. Symptomatic improvement occurred in 92% of patients based upon their visual analog pain score and their Prolo score [16].

Percutaneous and Endoscopic Discectomy

Overall, posterior minimally invasive lumbar procedures can be divided into two broad categories: (1) posterolateral or transforaminal intradiscal procedures and (2) posterior minimal access extradiscal procedures [2]. All percutaneous discectomy techniques share in common the primary goal of removing a portion of the nucleus pulposus whether it be by heat ablation or laser energy via a small-bore cannula such that a symptomatic compressed nerve root is adequately decompressed. The first successful 'percutaneous nucleotomy' was reported by Hijikata et al. in 1989 [17, 18]. Numerous percutaneous techniques have been evaluated with level 3 evidence, including percutaneous nucleotomy [18–22], percutaneous laser disc decompression using the YAG laser [19–21], and percutaneous plasma discectomy ('nucleoplasty') using the Coblation Spine Wand (ArthroCare, Sunnyvale, Calif., USA) (fig. 1) [23–25].

Another technique known as intradiscal electrothermal annuloplasty (or 'IDET') (Smith & Nephew Endoscopy, Andover, Mass., USA) has been developed that involves the percutaneous insertion of a thermal resistance probe with controlled heating of the disc material. IDET was developed as a minimally invasive procedure for the treatment of pain due to degenerative disc disease [26]. The procedure has been used in the lumbar spine of patients who have failed conservative treatment regimens and who might otherwise be candidates for a spinal fusion procedure. There have been multiple level 3 peer-reviewed articles that have presented favorable clinical outcomes associated with the IDET procedure [27–33]. In addition, a randomized, double-blind, placebo-controlled trial evaluating the efficacy of IDET for the treatment of chronic discogenic low back pain with 6-month outcome data has been successfully performed and published [34].

More work has been published on percutaneous chemonucleolysis than any other percutaneous discectomy technique and level I and level II evidence supports its use [35–38]. A double-blind study reported by Gogan and Fraser [39] demonstrated that 80% of the chymopapain-treated patients considered the injections to be successful compared with 34% of the saline-treated group, at 10 years ($p = 0.0006$). Javid [40] reported the results of a comparison between

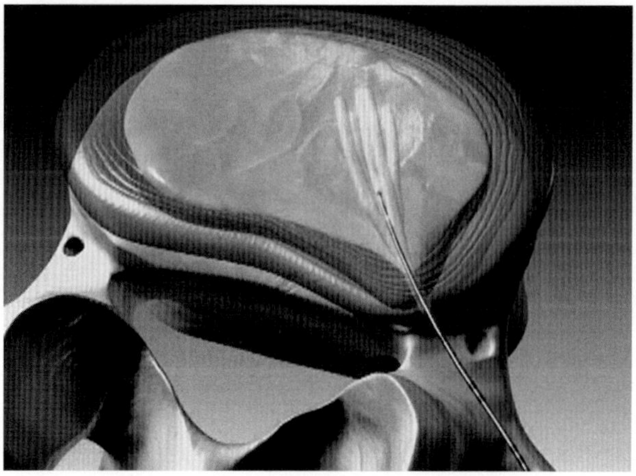

Fig. 1. The percutaneous plasma discectomy ('nucleoplasty') technique using the Coblation Spine Wand (ArthroCare) demonstrating the concept of intradiscal nucleus removal for symptomatic contained disc herniations.

laminectomy and chemonucleolysis, noting that 83% of the chemonucleolysis-treated patients and 76% of the laminectomy-treated patients demonstrated good results at 1 year.

Several mechanical means of decompressing the intervertebral disc space have been used for several decades. All of these techniques share in common a posterolateral approach to achieve the reduction of a herniated disc fragment to alleviate low back and/or radicular symptoms through a minimally invasive technique with minimum bony and soft tissue manipulation. The advent of high-resolution arthroscopes and video-assisted endoscopes made the direct visualized decompressions possible and safe. Evidence level 1 and 2 studies support the efficacy of arthroscopic disc surgery [41, 42]. Numerous evidence level 3 studies also support the efficacy of arthroscopic disc surgery [43].

In 1997, a microendoscopic discectomy system was introduced by Foley and Smith [44] to allow for the decompression of a symptomatic lumbar nerve root via an endoscopic approach. Unlike percutaneous approaches, the METRx system allows surgeons to address not only contained lumbar disc herniations, but also sequestered disc fragments and lateral recess stenosis. This technique has also been used for microendoscopic decompression of lumbar stenosis [12]. Three evidence level 3 studies [45–47] have been published. All three studies demonstrated greater than 92% excellent or good outcomes with a complication rate of 5% or less. The efficacy of this technique has been documented in a prospective multicenter trial [48]. These series also showed a significant reduction in operative time, reduced hospital stays, and return to work time compared to reports from the open discectomy literature.

Thoracoscopic Approaches

Thoracoscopic endoscopic procedures were first described by Kux [49] in 1951, who used urological endoscopes for the treatment of tuberculous disease. Thoracoscopic spinal surgery is a technique that provides full, direct access to the ventral thoracic spine. Class III evidence supports this technique for removing benign intrathoracic paraspinal neurogenic tumors, some corpectomies, spinal deformity correction, and central herniated thoracic discs. Its morbidity rate appears to be lower than that associated with open thoracotomy, and it improves patient comfort and cosmetic results and shortens recovery [50, 51]. Outcomes assessment was based upon patients' report of pain relief, mean operative time, length of hospitalization, blood loss, complications, and patients' willingness to repeat surgery under similar circumstances.

Sympathectomy for the treatment of hyperhydrosis and pain syndromes of the upper extremities has recently evolved from invasive open procedures to endoscopic procedures by taking advantage of minimally invasive thoracoscopic techniques [52]. There are multiple evidence level 5 studies that report successful outcomes using thoracoscopic techniques for minimally invasive thoracic sympathectomy in reducing overall procedure-related morbidity compared to previous open thoracotomy or posterior paraspinal approaches [53, 54]. These techniques have been further refined with reduced invasiveness using smaller and fewer incisions through biportal and uniportal exposure and simplified sympathectomy procedures to shorten hospital stay and further reduce morbidity [52, 55–59]. The class III evidence is based upon a binary response for outcomes assessment, evaluation of hospital length of stay, and the occurrence of complications [52, 57].

Thoracoscopic spinal surgery has been used with limited experience to achieve spinal decompression, reconstruction, and stabilization [2, 60]. Retrospectively evaluated level 5 data conclude that complete anterior thoracoscopically assisted reconstruction of thoracic and thoracolumbar fractures can be safely and effectively accomplished, thereby reducing the pain and morbidity associated with conventional thoracotomy and thoracolumbar approaches. The learning curve was felt by the authors to be quite steep. Video-assisted thoracic spine surgery demonstrated numerous benefits over open thoracotomy. These included decreased postoperative pain, faster recovery times, shorter hospital stays, less postoperative pulmonary complications, and reduction of shoulder girdle dysfunction [61, 62]. Such procedures require anterior spinal instrumentation systems specifically designed for endoscopic fixation.

Thoracolumbar Instrumentation

The minimally invasive placement of thoracolumbar instrumentation has followed the evolution of minimal access decompressive spinal surgery procedures. Traditional open posterior lumbar procedures result in significant iatrogenic injury to the dorsal musculoligamentous complex. Such procedures have been associated with significant long-term sequelae and complications. By reducing the amount of soft-tissue exposure needed at each step of the interbody fusion procedure, from discectomy through interbody graft placement to pedicle screw instrumentation, a minimally invasive percutaneous technique minimizes the amount of operative iatrogenic injury without sacrificing any of the goals of traditional open procedures [2]. The use of any of these techniques is supported only by class III evidence.

Foley designed the Sextant (Medtronic Sofamor Danek, Memphis, Tenn., USA) system for the expressed purpose of achieving a percutaneous pedicle screw rod fixation of the lumbar spine (fig. 2) [63]. The Pathfinder (Spinal Concepts, Austin, Tex., USA) is a more recent percutaneous pedicle instrumentation system that allows for multiple level instrumentation, compression, distraction and reduction of spondylolisthesis. Percutaneous lumbar pedicle screw instrumentation has been widely reported in a number of evidence level 5 studies [64, 65].

Direct visualization and concurrent posterolateral intertransverse fusion are not possible through these percutaneous systems. The ATAVI system (Endius, Plainville, Mass., USA) allows for the placement of pedicle screws directly through a minimal access tube (fig. 3). Similarly, the Aperture system (DePuy AcroMed, Johnson & Johnson, Rayham, Mass., USA) utilizes a specialized retractor system that seeks to minimize injury to the musculoligamentous complex. The drawback of more tissue dissection and manipulation of these two systems is offset by the ability to perform a wide range of procedures including decompression, discectomy, interbody fusion and grafting, and intertransverse onlay arthrodesis [2].

The anterior surgical approach to the lumbar spine offers itself to minimal access technology for interbody fusion and total disc replacement. Class III evidence supports the safety and efficacy of microsurgical anterior approaches [66, 67]. A laparoscopic approach to the anterior lumbar spine has been described as a safe and effective surgical technique [68, 69]. Given the long postoperative recovery time associated with a standard open approach, the

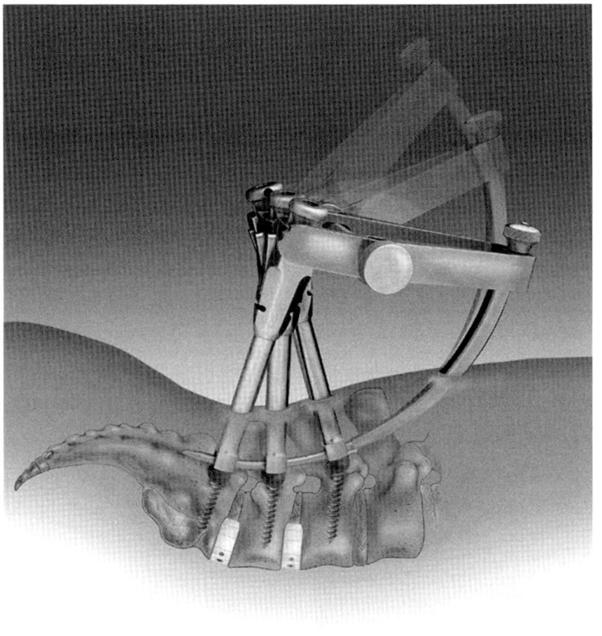

Fig. 2. The Sextant system for percutaneous pedicle screw instrumentation placement (Medtronic Sofamor Danek) utilizes cannulated polyaxial screws that are connected via a constrained arc-type rod inserter.

laparoscopic approach has been reported for the anterior lumbar interbody fusion procedure. The technique has been demonstrated to be safe and effective using the outcomes of blood loss, length of hospital stay, rate of fusion, and complications [70]. Evidence level 4 and 5 studies [71] demonstrate few advantages over a mini-open retroperitoneal approach [72] and an associated high complication rate [73].

Vertebroplasty and Kyphoplasty

Percutaneous acrylic vertebroplasty for the treatment of spinal compression fractures was developed in France and first described in 1987 [74]. This procedure uses a large-bore needle to percutaneously access a fractured vertebral body, inject bone cement, and thereby stabilize and reinforce the remaining bone structure. The technique is used to treat both osteoporotic as well as

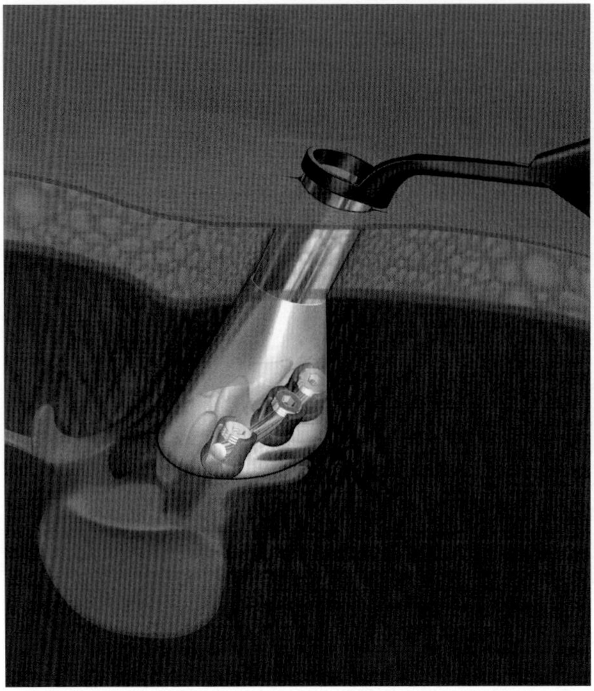

Fig. 3. The ATAVI system (Endius) allows for direct visualization and placement of pedicle screws through an expanding tubular portal.

pathologic compression fractures. Multiple evidence level 4 and 5 observational cohort studies have been published assessing vertebroplasty [75–80]. The primary outcome measure for these studies has been pain reduction; most series report a greater than 90% success rate using this outcome measure. However, most of these studies suffer from extremely short follow-up and lack of valid outcome instruments to assess true improvement in patient quality of life after the procedure.

The kyphoplasty procedure differs from vertebroplasty in that it attempts to address the limitation of little or no restoration of vertebral body height with stabilization. The inflatable bone tamp by Kyphon (Sunnyvale, Calif., USA) is placed through a cannula into the vertebral body and inflated with a balloonplasty technique to not only create a focal cavity to fill with cement, but also to attempt reexpansion of the vertebral body and thus regain height (fig. 4). Multiple evidence level 4 and 5 studies using validated outcome instruments

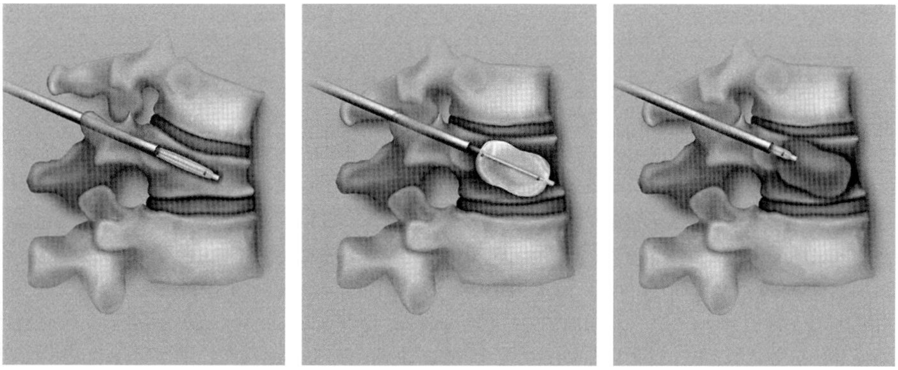

Fig. 4. The kyphoplasty technique (Kyphon) involves the placement of an inflatable bone tamp through a cannula into the vertebral body and inflation with a balloon-plasty technique that allows for vertebral body height restoration and the creation of a focal cavity to fill with cement.

support the use of kyphoplasty as being both safe and effective [81–86]. The scientific evidence for successful patient outcomes related to the kyphoplasty technique is better supported in the literature than for vertebroplasty, although the two techniques have not been properly directly compared in a single trial to date.

Stereotactic Spinal Radiosurgery and Radiotherapy

Given the success of radiosurgery to treat a variety of intracranial lesions, there has been an increased interest in the use of high doses of radiation to treat spinal lesions in this minimally invasive fashion. Current image-guided stereotactic radiosurgery/radiotherapy systems such as the CyberKnife (Accuray, Sunnyvale, Calif., USA) and the Novalis system (BrainLAB, Munich, Germany) and Portal Vision software (Varian Medical System, Palo Alto, Calif., USA) now allow for spinal stereotactic radiosurgery and intensity-modulated radiotherapy [87–91]. With adequate long-term safety follow-up, class III data has determined that spinal radiosurgery and radiotherapy are safe and effective alternatives to open surgery for a variety of both benign and malignant spinal tumors. Outcomes have focused on improvement in pain scores, safety, and improvement in both radiculopathy and myelopathy related to tumor compression [87, 88].

Conclusions

Minimally invasive surgical decompression, arthrodesis, and instrumentation techniques are now being applied in a wide variety of percutaneous, laparoscopic and minimal access procedures ranging from discectomy to multilevel laminectomy, to posterolateral in situ fusion, to posterior lumbar interbody fusion and transforaminal lumbar interbody fusion. It is crucial, however, to realize that there is little to no longitudinal long-term data on these procedures to document their efficacy, indications, limitations and complications as compared to standard open techniques [2]. As such, evidence level 1 and 2 randomized trials are required to ultimately prove these benefits and also to justify the sometimes significant increased costs of these minimally invasive surgical procedures.

It is clear that the present wave of minimally invasive surgery procedures represents an important shift in the practice of contemporary spinal surgery. With subsequent advances in biological, regenerative, dynamic stabilization, and radiation-targeting technologies, the access and instrumentation techniques developed for present-day minimally invasive surgical procedures will also form the basis for delivering these future technologies to the spine with a minimum of iatrogenic injury [2]. Evidence-based medicine standards will constantly struggle to stay abreast of this quickly advancing subspecialty.

References

1 Jaikumar S, Kim DH, Kam AC: History of minimally invasive spine surgery. Neurosurgery 2002;51:1–14.
2 Khoo LT, Gravori T: Minimally invasive posterior spinal decompression and fusion procedures. SpineLine 2003;5:9.
3 McCormick PC: Preface. Neurosurgery 2002;51:v–vi.
4 Fessler RG: Foreward. Neurosurgery 2002;51:iii–iv.
5 Gerszten PC: Outcomes research: a review. Neurosurgery 1998;43:1148–1151.
6 King J, Joseph T: Quality of life assessment with the medical outcomes study short form-36 among patients with cervical spondylotic myelopathy. Neurosurgery 2003;52:113–121.
7 Daltroy L, Cats-Baril W, Katz J, et al: The North American spine society lumbar spine outcome assessment instrument: reliability and validity tests. Spine 1996;21:741–749.
8 Fairbank J, Cooper J, Davies J, et al: The Oswestry low back pain disability questionnaire. Physiotherapy 1980;66:271–273.
9 Haines SJ: Evidence-based neurosurgery. Neurosurgery 2003;52:36–47.
10 Lohr KN: Outcome measurement: concepts and questions. Inquiry 1988;25:37–50.
11 Benzel EC: Preface. Neurosurgery 2002;51:vi.
12 Fessler R, Guiot B, Khoo L: A minimally invasive technique for decompression of the lumbar spine. Spine 2002;27:432–438.
13 Murphey F, Simmons JC, Brunson B: Surgical treatment of laterally ruptured cervical discs: review of 648 cases, 1939–1972. J Neurosurg 1973;38:679–683.
14 Zeidman S, Ducker T: Posterior cervical laminoforaminotomy for radiculopathy: review of 172 cases. Neurosurgery 1993;33:356–362.

15 Adamson TE: Microendoscopic posterior cervical laminoforaminotomy for unilateral radiculopathy: results of a new technique in 100 cases. J Neurosurg Spine 2001;95:51–57.
16 Fessler RG, Khoo LT: Minimally invasive cervical microendoscopic foraminotomy: an initial clinical experience. Neurosurgery 2002;51:37–45.
17 Hijikata S: Percutaneous nucleotomy: a new concept technique and 12 years' experience. Clin Orthop 1989;238:9–23.
18 Maroon J, Onik G, Vidovich D: Percutaneous discectomy for lumbar disc herniation. Neurosurg Clin N Am 1993;4:125–134.
19 Casper G, Hartman V, Mullins L: Percutaneous laser disc decompression with the holmium: YAG laser. J Clin Laser Med Surg 1995;13:195–203.
20 Choy D: Percutaneous laser disc decompression (PLDD): twelve years' experience with 752 procedures in 518 patients. J Clin Laser Med Surg 1998;16:325–331.
21 Gangi A, Dietemann J, Ide C, et al: Percutaneous laser disk decompression under CT and fluoroscopic guidance: indications, techniques and clinical experience. Radiographics 1996;16:89–96.
22 Kotilainen E, Valtonen S: Long-term outcome of patients who underwent percutaneous nucleotomy for lumbar disc herniation: results after a mean follow-up of 5 years. Acta Neurochir (Wien) 1998;140:108–113.
23 Andreula C, Muto M, Leonardi M: Interventional spine procedures. Eur J Radiol 2004;50: 112–119.
24 Chen Y, Lee S, Saenz Y, et al: Histologic findings of disc, end plant and neural elements after coblation of nucleus pulposus: an experimental nucleoplasty study. Spine 2003;3:466–470.
25 Dworkin G: Advanced concepts in interventional spine care. J Am Osteopath Assoc 2002;102: 8–11.
26 Heary RF: Intradiscal electrothermal annuloplasty: the IDET procedure; in Resnick DK, Haid RW Jr: Surgical Management of Low Back Pain. The American Association of Neurological Surgeons, Rolling Meadows, 2001, pp 143–150.
27 Derby R, Eek B, Chen Y, et al: Intradiscal electrothermal annuloplasty (IDET): a novel approach for treating chronic discogenic back pain. Neuromodulation 2000;3:82–88.
28 Freedman BA, Cohen SP, Kuklo TR, et al: Intradiscal electrothermal therapy (IDET) for chronic low back pain in active-duty soldiers: 2-year follow-up. Spine J 2003;3:502–509.
29 Gerszten PC, Welch WC, McGrath PM, et al: A prospective outcomes study of patients undergoing intradiscal electrothermy (IDET) for chronic low back pain. Pain Physician 2002;5:360–364.
30 Karasek M, Bogduk N: Twelve-month follow-up of a controlled trial on intradiscal thermal annuloplasty for back pain due to internal disc disrupture. Spine 2000;25:2601–2607.
31 McGraw JK, Silber JS: Intradiscal electrothermal therapy for the treatment of discogenic back pain. Appl Radiol 2001;30:11–16.
32 Saal JA, Saal JS: Intradiscal electrothermal treatment for chronic discogenic low back pain: a prospective outcome study with minimum 1-year follow-up. Spine 2000;25:2622–2627.
33 Wetzel FT, McNally TA, Phillips FM: Intradiscal electrothermal therapy used to manage chronic discogenic low back pain new directions and interventions. Spine 2002;27:2621–2626.
34 Pauza K, Howell S, Dreyfuss P, et al: A randomized, placebo controlled trial of intradiscal electrothermal therapy for the treatment of discogenc low back pain. Spine J 2004;4:27–35.
35 Kim Y-S, Chin D-K, Cho Y-E, et al: Predictors of successful outcome for lumbar chemonucleolysis: analysis of 3,000 cases during the past 14 years. Neurosurgery 2002;51:123–128.
36 Mansfield F, Polivy K, Boyd R, et al: Long-term results of chymopapain injections. Clin Orthop 1996;206:67–69.
37 Maroon J, Abla A: Microdiscectomy versus chemonucleolysis. Neurosurgery 1985;16:644–649.
38 Tregonning G, Transfelds E, McCulloch J, et al: Chymopapain versus conventional surgery for lumbar disc herniation: 10-year results of treatment. J Bone Joint Surg Br 1991;73B:481–486.
39 Gogan W, Fraser R: Chymopapain: a 10-year, double blind study. Spine 1992;17:388–394.
40 Javid M: Chemonucleolysis versus laminectomy: a cohort comparison of effectiveness and charges. Spine 1995;20:2016–2022.
41 Hermantin F, Peters TM, Quartararo L, et al: A prospective, randomized study comparing the results of open discectomy with those of video-assisted arthroscopic microdiscectomy. J Bone Joint Surg Am 1999;81A:958–965.

42 Mayer H, Brock M: Percutaneous endoscopic discectomy: surgical technique and preliminary results compared to microsurgical discectomy. J Neurosurg 1993;78:216–225.
43 Kambin P: Arthroscopic microdiscectomy. Arthroscopy 1992;8:287–295.
44 Foley K, Smith M: Microendoscopic discectomy. Tech Neurosurg 1997;3:301–307.
45 Foley K, Smith M, Rampersaud Y: Microendoscopic approach to far-lateral lumbar disc herniation. Neurosurg Focus 1999;7:article 5.
46 Hilton D: Microdiscectomy with a minimally invasive tubular retractor; in Perez-Cruet M, Fessler R (eds): Outpatient Spinal Surgery. St Louis, Quality Medical Publishing, 2002, pp 159–170.
47 Perez-Cruet M, Foley K, Isaacs R, et al: Microendoscopic lumbar discectomy: technical note. Neurosurgery 2002;51:129–136.
48 Foley K, Smith M, Rampersaud Y: Microendoscopic discectomy; in Schmidek H (ed): Operative Neurosurgical Techniques: Indications, Methods, and Results. Philadelphia, Saunders, 2000.
49 Kux E: The endoscopic approach to the vegetative nervous system and its therapeutic possibilities. Dis Chest 1951;20:139–147.
50 Dickman C, Rosenthal D, Karahalios DG, Paramore C, et al: Thoracic vertebrectomy and reconstruction using a microsurgical thorascopic approach. Neurosurgery 1996;38:279–293.
51 Han PP, Kenny K, Dickman CA: Thoracoscopic approaches to the thoracic spine: experience with 241 surgical procedures. Neurosurgery 2002;51:88–95.
52 Johnson JP, Patel NP: Uniportal and biportal endoscopic thoracic sympathectomy. Neurosurgery 2002;51:79–83.
53 Drott C, Gothberg G, Claes G: Endoscopic procedures of the upper thoracic sympathetic chain: a review. Arch Surg 1993;128:237–241.
54 Kux E: Thoracic endoscopic sympathectomy in palmar and axillary hyperhidrosis. Arch Surg 1978;113:264–266.
55 Dumont P, Hamm A, Skrobala D, et al: Bilateral thoracoscopy for sympathectomy in the treatment of hyperhidrosis. Eur J Surg 1997;11:774–775.
56 Lardinois D, Ris H: Minimally invasive video-endoscopic sympathectomy by use of a transaxillary single port approach. Eur J Cardiothorac Surg 2002;21:67–70.
57 Lin T-S, Kuo S-J, Chou M-C: Uniportal endoscopic thoracic sympathectomy for treatment of palmar and axillary hyperhidrosis: analysis of 2000 cases. Neurosurgery 2002;51:84–87.
58 Reardon P, Preciado A, Scarborough T, et al: Outpatient endoscopic thoracic sympathectomy using 2-mm instruments. Surg Endosc 1999;13:1139–1142.
59 Wahlig JB, Welch WC, Weigel TL, et al: Microinvasive transaxillary thoracoscopic sympathectomy: technical note. Neurosurgery 2000;46:1254–1258.
60 Horn EM, Henn JS, Lemole GM Jr, et al: Thoracoscopic placement of dual-rod instrumentation in thoracic spinal trauma. Neurosurgery 2004;54:1150–1154.
61 Beisse R, Potulski M, Buhren V: Endoscopic techniques for the management of spinal trauma. Eur J Trauma 2001;27:275–291.
62 Regan J, Mack M, Picetti G 3rd: A comparison of video-assisted thoracoscopic surgery (VATS) with open thoracotomy in thoracic spinal surgery. Today's Ther Trends 1994;11:203–218.
63 Foley K, Gupta S, Justis J, et al: Percutaneous pedicle screw fixation of the lumbar spine. Neurosurg Focus 2001;10:1–8.
64 Lowery G, Kulkarni S: Posterior percutaneous spine instrumentation. Eur Spine J 2000;9:216–130.
65 Wiesner L, Kothe R, Ruther W: Anatomic evaluation of two different techniques for the percutaneous insertion of pedicle screws in the lumbar spine. Spine 1999;24:1599–1603.
66 Mathews H, Evans M, Molligan H, et al: Laparoscopic discectomy with anterior lumbar interbody fusion. Spine 1995;20:1797–1802.
67 Mayer HM, Wiechert K: Microsurgical anterior approaches to the lumbar spine for interbody fusion and total disc replacement. Neurosurgery 2002;51:159–165.
68 Lieberman I, Willsher P, Litwin D, et al: Transperitoneal laparoscopic exposure for lumbar interbody fusion. Spine 2000;25:509–515.
69 Regan J, McAfee PC, Guyer R, et al: Laparoscopic fusion of the lumbar spine in a multicenter series of the first 34 patients. Surg Laparosc Endosc 1996;6:459–468.
70 Liu JC, Ondra SL, Angelos P, et al: Is laparoscopic anterior lumbar interbody fusion a useful minimally invasive procedure? Neurosurgery 2002;51:155–158.

71 Regan JJ, Yuan H, McAfee PC: Laparoscopic fusion of the lumbar spine: minimally invasive spine surgery: a prospective multicenter study evaluating open and laparoscopic lumbar fusion. Spine 1999;24:402–411.
72 Dewald C, Millikan K, Hammerberg K, et al: An open, minimally invasive approach to the lumbar spine. Am Surg 1999;65:61–68.
73 McAfee P, Regan J, Zdeblick TA, et al: The incidence of complications in endoscopic anterior thoracolumbar spinal reconstructive surgery. Spine 1995;20:1623–1632.
74 Galibert P, Deramond H: Note préliminaire sur le traitement des angiomes vertébraux par vertébroplastie acrylique percutanée. Neurochirurgie 1987;33:166–168.
75 Barr JD, Barr MS, Lemley TJ, et al: Percutaneous vertebroplasty for pain relief and spinal stabilization. Spine 2000;25:923–928.
76 Cortet B, Cotten A, Boutry N, et al: Percutaneous vertebroplasty in the treatment of osteoporotic vertebral compression fractures: an open prospective study. J Rheumatol 1999;26:2222–2228.
77 Deramond H, Depriester C, Galibert P, et al: Percutaneous vertebroplasty with polymethylmethacrylate. Radiol Clin North Am 1998;36:533–546.
78 Jensen ME, Evans AJ, Mathis JM, et al: Percutaneous polymethylmethacrylate vertebroplasty in the treatment of osteoporotic vertebral body compression fractures: technical aspects. Am J Neuroradiol 1997;18:1897–1904.
79 Peters KR, Guiot BH, Martin PA, et al: Vertebroplasty for osteoporotic compression fracture: current practice and evolving techniques. Neurosurgery 2002;51:96–103.
80 Wong W, Reiley MA, Garfin S: Vertebroplasty/kyphoplasty. J Womens Imaging 2000;2:117–124.
81 Berlemann U, Franz T, Orler R, Heini PF: Kyphoplasty for treatment of osteoporotic vertebral fractures: a prospective non-randomized study. Eur Spine J 2004;13:496–501.
82 Coumans J: Kyphoplasty for vertebral compression fractures: 1-year clinical outcomes from a prospective study. J Neurosurg 2003;99:44–50.
83 Dudeney S: Kyphoplasty in the treatment of osteolytic vertebral compression fractures as a result of multiple myeloma. J Clin Oncol 2002;20:2382–2387.
84 Ledlie J, Renfro M: Balloon kyphoplasty: one-year outcomes in vertebral body height restoration, chronic pain and activity levels. J Neurosurg Spine 2003;98:36–42.
85 Lieberman I, Dudeney S, Reinhardt M: Initial outcome and efficacy of 'kyphoplasty' in the treatment of painful osteoporotic vertebral compression fractures. Spine 2001;26:1631–1638.
86 Rhyne A 3rd, Banit D, Laxer E, Odum S, Nussman D: Kyphoplaty: report of eighty-two thoracolumbar osteoporotic vertebral fractures. J Orthop Trauma 2004;18:294–299.
87 Bilsky MH: Intensity-modulated stereotactic radiotherapy or paraspinal tumors: a preliminary report. Neurosurgery 2004;54:823–831.
88 Gerszten PC, Ozhasoglu C, Burton S, et al: CyberKnife frameless stereotactic radiosurgery for spinal lesions: clinical experience in 125 cases. Neurosurgery 2004;55:89–99.
89 Klimo P Jr, Schmidt MH: Surgical management of spinal metastases. Oncologist 2004;9:188–196.
90 Ryu S, Yin FF, Rock J, et al: Image-guided and intensity-modulated radiosurgery for patients with spinal metastasis. Cancer 2003;97:2013–2018.
91 Ryu SI, Chang SD, Kim DH, et al: Image-guided hypo-fractionated stereotactic radiosurgery to spinal lesions. Neurosurgery 2001;49:838–846.

Peter C. Gerszten, MD, MPH
Department of Neurological Surgery, Presbyterian University Hospital
Suite B-400, 200 Lothrop St.
Pittsburgh, PA 15213 (USA)
Tel. +1 412 647 0958, Fax +1 412 647 0989, E-Mail gersztenpc@upmc.edu

Pollock BE (ed): Guiding Neurosurgery by Evidence.
Prog Neurol Surg. Basel, Karger, 2006, vol 19, pp 152–170

An Evidence-Based Medicine Review of Stereotactic Radiosurgery

Bruce E. Pollock

Departments of Neurological Surgery and Radiation Oncology,
Mayo Clinic College of Medicine, Rochester, Minn., USA

Abstract

Background: Stereotactic radiosurgery has been increasingly utilized to manage a wide variety of indications including vascular malformations, benign and malignant tumors, and functional disorders. **Methods:** Review of the recent literature on stereotactic radiosurgery by evidence-based standards. **Results:** The vast majority of published papers on stereotactic radiosurgery is of rather poor quality (level 3 or below). Two studies provide level 1 evidence showing an improvement in local tumor control or survival for patients with 1–3 brain metastases having radiosurgery in conjunction with whole brain radiation therapy when compared to patients having whole brain radiation therapy alone. One randomized trial found no improvement in facial pain outcomes for trigeminal neuralgia patients having a longer segment of the nerve irradiated. **Conclusion:** For a variety of reasons it is unlikely that randomized clinical trials will be performed to evaluate the clinical usefulness of stereotactic radiosurgery. Nonetheless, the preponderance of level 3 information supports the role of radiosurgery as either an adjunct or alternative to surgical resection or fractionated radiation therapy.

Lars Leksell [1, 2] of the Karolinska Institute in Stockholm, Sweden conceived the concept of stereotactic radiosurgery (SRS) as a less invasive method to create closed skull, ablative lesions, primarily for functional procedures. SRS combined stereotactic localization techniques developed in neurosurgery with radiation physics to distribute energy (X-rays, gamma rays, protons) to an imaging defined target. As described by Leksell, the radiation was delivered in a single procedure (dose) to the intended target with a steep dose falloff. During the 1960s and early 1970s, Leksell and his colleagues, primarily radiobiologist Börje Larsson, tried a variety of devices and they eventually decided that a fixed cobalt-60 device was the best solution and the original Gamma Knife® (Elekta Instruments, Norcross, Ga., USA) was developed. Inspired by the work of Leksell, other investigators, including Jacob Fabrikant, Raymond Kjellberg, Ken Winston, Jay Loeffler, Osvaldo Betti, Federico Colombo, William Freidman, and Frank Bova (to name only a few), were working simultaneously on systems that used heavy particles from cyclotrons or X-rays from modified linear accelerators as the energy sources for radiosurgery.

Progress in both neuroimaging and dose planning software significantly improved patient outcomes after radiosurgery. Radiosurgery is now commonly accepted as the best management for many patients with brain tumors and vascular malformations. It is a multidisciplinary surgical procedure that requires dedicated technology and facilities. Whereas once SRS existed only in academic centers, today more than 200 hospitals and outpatient facilities perform radiosurgery in the United States alone. It is estimated that more than 50,000 patients underwent radiosurgery last year. SRS is now an important part in the training of neurosurgical and radiation oncology residents.

This chapter will review the published information on radiosurgery of vascular malformations, tumors, and functional disorders according to evidence-based medicine (EBM) guidelines. Specifically, the papers covered will refer to single-session procedures (radiosurgery) as opposed to procedures utilizing image-guided, multiple-session radiation delivery (stereotactic radiation therapy) [3].

Application of EBM to Radiosurgery

EBM is the conscientious, explicit and judicious use of the current best evidence in making decisions about the care of individual patients [4]. In the late 1970s, Suzanne Fletcher and Dave Sackett generated the idea of 'levels of evidence' to rank the validity of evidence of preventive healthcare measures and linked them to 'grades of recommendations' for different interventions [5]. Briefly, the most valid information (level 1) is obtained when a particular therapy has been studied with multiple randomized clinical trials (RCT) with little variation in the direction or magnitude of the results. In situations where consistent level 1 studies exist, a grade A recommendation can be made for that particular therapy. Levels 2, 3, 4 and 5 refer to cohort studies, case-control series, case series, and expert opinions, respectively. Grade B recommendation can be made with consistent level 2 or 3 studies (or extrapolation from level 1 studies), grade C recommendations can be made from level 4 studies (or extrapolation from level 2 or 3 studies), and grade D recommendations can be made from level 5 studies (or inconsistent or inconclusive studies of any level). By incorporating the best available external evidence together with our clinical expertise and consideration of an individual's life situation and preferences, a physician is able to employ an EBM practice.

A variety of reasons exist that limit the practical ability of neurosurgeons to perform RCTs for each situation. First, and particularly relevant to neurosurgery, is that the condition of interest may be rare. Even in settings were the magnitude of effectiveness between different treatments is large, a sufficient number of patients must be enrolled to show this difference in a statistically meaningful way. Second, for benign tumors such as meningiomas or vestibular schwannomas (VS), the success of an operation in preventing tumor recurrence or progression may not be evident for 10 or more years after surgery. Thus, the information derived from case series (level 4 evidence) may be the best available data to base clinical decision making for patients with benign tumors and extended life expectancies. Third, and particularly relevant to radiosurgery, is the fact that few patients are willing to participate in randomized trials in which one group has open surgery whereas the other undergoes radiosurgery. In fact, more and more patients have decided based upon their own research before an official consultation with a neurosurgeon that they want one particular procedure, and they seek out physicians and centers with expertise in that operation. For such self-educated patients, the concept of allowing chance to determine whether they undergo a craniotomy with a several day hospital stay or a procedure done as an outpatient under local anesthesia is inconceivable. So although an RCT comparing outcomes after surgical resection and radiosurgery for VS or brain metastases would likely yield critical information, the 'trial ability' of such proposed studies is low. For these and many other reasons, clinicians most often have to base their decision making on rather poor quality evidence.

Benign Tumors

SRS has become an accepted treatment option for patients with meningiomas [6–13], VS [14–23], non-VS [24–27], and pituitary adenomas [28–36]. Each year, thousands of patients worldwide undergo radiosurgery for these benign tumor types. In many respects, patients with benign tumors are ideal candidates for radiosurgery. First, unlike malignant gliomas, these tumors rarely invade the adjacent tissue and therefore focused approaches such as radiosurgery can be used to completely treat the entire tumor burden. Second, benign tumors are typically well visualized by magnetic resonance imaging (MRI). This permits a clear delineation between the tumor and nearby structures so unnecessary radiation exposure can be minimized. Third, radiosurgery of benign tumors makes radiobiologic sense [37]. For benign tumors, both the target and the adjacent nervous system act as late responding tissues due to their slow rate of proliferation. Consequently, dose fractionation adds little theoretical benefit compared to conformal, single fraction radiation delivery.

Despite these factors supporting benign tumor radiosurgery, the available papers on radiosurgery of benign tumors had primarily level 4 evidence regarding its relative effectiveness compared to other treatments. For example, Nikolopoulos and O'Donoghue [38] reviewed papers published in English over 23 years on the management VS patients. Of the 111 papers examined, 18% (20 studies) pertained to VS radiosurgery. Overall, 91% of the papers had either level 3 or 4 evidence; no paper provided level 1 or 2 evidence to support surgical resection, radiosurgery, or observation. They concluded that the overall quality of data available on VS management was poor, and that efforts should be made to improve the quality of evidence on this topic. Unfortunately, the situation for radiosurgery of meningiomas, nonacoustic schwannomas, and pituitary adenomas is no better with the overwhelming number of studies being individual case series (level 4 evidence (table 1)).

Vestibular Schwannomas

The best management of patients with VS is one of the most controversial topics in neurosurgery [39–41]. Four studies have used a retrospective cohort methodology to compare outcomes after radiosurgery to surgical resection for VS patients [17, 20, 22, 23]. Pollock et al. [20] compared 87 patients with unilateral, unoperated VS with a mean diameter of 3 cm or less managed during 1990 and 1991 at the University of Pittsburgh. The patients having surgical resection were younger (51 vs. 62 years, $p < 0.001$); tumor sizes were similar. At a median follow-up of 36 months, patients having radiosurgery were more likely to have normal facial movement and preservation of 'useful hearing'. Hospital length of stay, return to independent functioning, and direct treatment charges were less with radiosurgery ($p < 0.001$). Van Roijen et al. [23] compared 53 VS patients having surgical resection at the University Hospital Rotterdam to 92 patients having radiosurgery at the Karolinska Institute in Sweden. Both patient groups were treated from 1990 to 1995. Although the inclusion criteria were similar in both groups (no prior treatment, unilateral tumor, and extrameatal diameter less than 3 cm), it is not stated whether the patients were consecutively treated. The response rate to the mailed questionnaire was 92% for both groups. Overall, radiosurgery was more cost-effective with regard to both direct and indirect costs. Using the Short-Form 36 to measure activities of daily living, patients having radiosurgery had higher scores in the physical function ($p < 0.05$), role physical ($p < 0.02$) and mental health ($p < 0.01$) domains. Radiosurgical patients also scored higher according to the EuroQol classification compared to the microsurgery group (0.89 vs. 0.77, $p < 0.01$).

Table 1. Levels of evidence for different radiosurgical indications

Indication	Comparison group	References	Best evidence	Comments
Benign tumors				
Vestibular schwannoma	surgical resection	[17, 20, 22, 23]	level 3	radiosurgery has better cranial nerve preservation rates
	SRT	[42, 43]	level 3	similar results for tumor control, trigeminal and facial nerve function; conflicting results for hearing preservation
Meningioma	surgical resection	[10]	level 3	radiosurgery had similar tumor control as Simpson Grade 1 resection; lower complication rate
Pituitary adenoma (acromegaly)	radiation therapy	[29]	level 3	radiosurgery had higher rate of endocrine cure
Malignant tumors				
Brain metastases	WBRT alone versus WBRT and SRS	[50, 70]	level 1	radiosurgery improved local tumor control; improved survival for patients with 1 tumor and for selected patients with 2 or 3 tumors
	surgical resection	[67–69]	level 3	conflicting results; one study showed survival better with resection; two studies [68, 69] had no difference in survival or tumor control
Gliomas	SRS+XRT+BCNU versus XRT+BCNU	[64]	level 1	SRS provided no improvement in survival or tumor control
	SRS as adjuvant therapy	[60–63]	level 4	potential survival benefit for selected patients
Vascular malformations				
AVM	observation	[71–74]	level 4	radiosurgery improves outcomes for majority of patients with small AVMs
CM	observation	[83–87]	level 4	hemorrhage rate appears to decline after latency interval; controversial

Functional				
Trigeminal neuralgia	high dose versus low dose	[91, 94, 95]	level 4	improved facial pain outcomes with higher doses
	one-shot versus two-shot	[90]	level 1	no improvement in facial pain results; power of study?
Temporal lobe epilepsy	temporal lobe resection	[99]	level 4	SRS has similar seizure-free rate compared to surgical resection

BCNU = 1,3-Bis(2-chloroethyl)-N-nitrosourea; XRT = fractionated radiation therapy.

Karpinos et al. [17] reviewed 96 patients with unilateral VS having radiosurgery or microsurgery from 1993 to 2000 at Memorial Hospital in Houston, Tex., USA. Patients having surgery were younger and had larger tumors compared to the radiosurgery group. Also, the microsurgical group had a longer median follow-up (48 vs. 24 months). In this comparison, radiosurgery was more effective at preservation of measurable hearing (58 vs. 14%, $p = 0.01$), and had lower rates of trigeminal (12 vs. 22%, $p < 0.01$) and facial neuropathies (0 vs. 35%, $p < 0.01$). Patients having microsurgery had longer hospital stays (2–16 vs. 1–2 days, $p < 0.01$) and more perioperative complications (48 vs. 5%, $p < 0.01$). Regis et al. [22] compared 97 VS patients having radiosurgery from 1992 to 1998 with 110 VS patients having surgical resection from 1983 to 1990 at the Timone Hospital in Marseille, France. Patients had to have unilateral tumors and no previous therapy for their VS. For statistical purposes, only patients with small- to medium-sized tumors (excluding purely intracanalicular and large tumors with brainstem displacement) were included. In this study, more men had radiosurgery (46 vs. 35%) and patients having radiosurgery were older (61 vs. 52 years). Using their own questionnaire and other objective data, new facial weakness was more common in the surgical group (37 vs. 0%). For patients with Gardner-Robertson class 1 hearing before treatment, preservation of class 1 or 2 hearing was more common in the radiosurgery group (70 vs. 38%). The mean time away from work was 7 days after radiosurgery and 130 days after surgical resection. The data available to compare radiosurgery and surgical resection in these four papers remains rather poor quality (level 3). However, the results in each study are consistent and show that in short-term follow-up, radiosurgery provides better functional outcomes than surgical resection for patients with unilateral, unoperated small- to medium-sized VS.

Two studies have compared the results of SRS to fractionated stereotactic radiotherapy (SRT) [42, 43]. Andrews et al. [42] reviewed 125 VS patients having radiosurgery ($n = 69$) or fractionated SRT ($n = 56$) from 1994 to 2000. The tumor margin dose for radiosurgery was 12 Gy; patients having SRT received a total dose of 50.4 Gy delivered in 28 fractions. The mean follow-up was just over 2 years in both groups. No difference was noted in tumor control, new trigeminal deficits, or new facial weakness. Patients having SRT were more likely to retain functional hearing compared to patients having radiosurgery. Meijer et al. [43] compared VS patients having either fractionated SRT (either 4 or 5 Gy $\times$ 5 fractions) of linac-based radiosurgery (10 or 12.5 Gy at 80% isodose line) between 1992 and 2000. Interestingly, patients were assigned to SRT if they had teeth ($n = 80$), whereas patients without teeth who could not use their relocatable stereotactic guide underwent radiosurgery using a conventional stereotactic headframe ($n = 49$). Patients having radiosurgery were older (63 vs. 49 years, $p = 0.001$); tumor sizes were similar between the groups. At a mean follow-up of 33 months, there was no difference in 5-year tumor control, facial movement, or hearing preservation. Patients having radiosurgery were more likely to develop new facial numbness (8 vs. 2%, $p < 0.05$). Therefore, much like the comparisons of surgical resection and radiosurgery for patients with VS, the best available information to compare radiosurgery and SRT for VS patients is level 3 evidence. The two papers on this topic show that patient outcomes are essentially equivalent over a short follow-up interval. With regard to hearing preservation, the results were conflicting with one paper showing higher rates of hearing preservation with SRT [42], whereas the other found similar hearing outcomes [43].

Meningiomas

Only one study has compared the results of radiosurgery to surgical resection for patients with intracranial meningiomas [10]. Similar to the VS comparison papers, Pollock et al. employed a retrospective cohort design to compare surgical resection and radiosurgery as the primary management for adult patients with benign meningiomas with an average tumor diameter of less than 35 mm. Between 1990 and 1997, 198 patients met these criteria and were analyzed for tumor recurrence or progression. The mean follow-up was 64 months. Tumor resections per Simpson grade were 1 (n = 57, 42%), 2 (n = 57, 42%), or 3–4 (n = 22, 16%). The mean margin and maximum radiation doses at radiosurgery were 17.7 and 34.9 Gy, respectively. Tumor recurrence/progression was more frequent in the surgical resection group (12%) compared to the radiosurgical group (2%; $p = 0.04$). No difference was detected in the 3- and 7-year actuarial progression-free survival (PFS) for patients having Simpson Grade 1 resections (100 and 96%) or radiosurgery (100 and 95%; $p = 0.94$). Radiosurgery provided a higher PFS rate compared to patients having Simpson Grade 2 (3- and 7-year PFS, 91 and 82%; $p < 0.05$) or Grade 3–4 resection (3- and 7-year PFS, 68 and 34%; $p < 0.001$). Subsequent tumor treatments were more common after surgical resection (15 vs. 3%, $p = 0.02$). Complications occurred in 10% of patients after radiosurgery compared to 22% of patients having tumor resection ($p = 0.06$). Therefore, in this study, the PFS rate after radiosurgery was equivalent to a Simpson Grade 1 resection, and was superior to Grades 2 and 3–4. Therefore, this single study supports radiosurgery (level 3 evidence) as the preferred management for the majority of patients with small- to moderate-sized meningiomas without symptomatic mass effect.

Pituitary Adenomas

Landolt et al. [29] compared the results of radiosurgery to fractionated radiation therapy for patients with recurrent acromegaly after prior surgery. Fifty patients having fractionated radiation therapy (median dose, 40 Gy) from

1973 to 1992 were compared to 16 patients having radiosurgery (median tumor margin dose, 25 Gy) between 1994 and 1996. Patient demographics, tumor size, and pretreatment growth hormone and insulin-like growth factor I were similar between the two treatment groups. The follow-up interval of patients having radiation therapy was significantly longer (7.5 vs. 1.4 years, $p < 0.0001$). Patients having radiosurgery more commonly achieved biochemical remission ($p < 0.0001$); the mean time to endocrine normalization was 1.4 years after radiosurgery compared to 7.1 years after fractionated radiation therapy. Thus, similar to other studies comparing benign tumor radiosurgery to other treatment options, this single study supports radiosurgery (level 3 evidence) over fractionated radiation therapy for patients with recurrent acromegaly.

Malignant Tumors

SRS is especially attractive to patients with malignant brain tumors because of its minimally invasive nature and the fact that no recovery period is required after the procedure is completed. However, although numerous papers have examined the usefulness of radiosurgery for patients with brain metastases [44–59] and gliomas [60–65], the relative role that radiosurgery should play in the treatment of these two indications is likely to be quite different because of their distinct cellular architecture. Brain metastases typically are focal collections of malignant cells with a clear separation between the tumor and the adjacent brain. Conversely, gliomas are generally infiltrative with indistinct edges and regions of tumor mixed with brain. Moreover, brain metastases are well-visualized on gadolinium-enhanced MRI; high-grade gliomas are often made up of a combination of enhancing and nonenhancing regions. Therefore, it has become apparent that radiosurgery can be used as the primary management for many patients with brain metastases, whereas radiosurgery is most often employed as an adjunct to surgical resection, radiation therapy, and chemotherapy for glioma patients.

Brain Metastases

For many decades the standard of care for patients with metastatic brain disease was whole-brain radiation therapy (WBRT). Despite advances in the detection and treatment of brain metastases, the median survival for patients treated with WBRT alone is approximately 4–6 months, and tumor recurrence/progression is common if the patient survives more than 1 year. Radiosurgery has been used to improve local tumor control rates, and most studies have found that over 80% of tumors treated with radiosurgery do not progress. Other factors that make radiosurgery an attractive option are that multiple tumors can be treated in a single session, and tumors in deep brain locations who are considered poor candidates for surgical resection can be effectively and safely treated. Questions that remain unanswered regarding brain metastasis radiosurgery include the appropriate roles of WBRT and radiosurgery [58, 66], and the relative indications of surgical resection versus radiosurgery for patients with brain metastases [67–71].

Kondziolka et al. [50] performed an RCT of 27 patients to compare survival and tumor control for patients having WBRT or WBRT and radiosurgery. They found that combined WBRT and SRS significantly improved local tumor control for patients with r2–4 brain metastases compared to patients receiving WBRT alone. No difference was noted in patient survival, although a difference was detected between patients who had WBRT alone in comparison to patients who later had salvage SRS or those who had initial WBRT and SRS. Andrews and colleagues [70] recently reported a prospective randomized RTOG trial (RTOG 95-08) of WBRT versus WBRT plus radiosurgery for patients with 1–3 brain metastases. WBRT plus radiosurgery provided a survival advantage compared to WBRT alone in the following patient groups: (1) patients with a single brain metastasis, (2) patients with 2 or 3 metastases and RPA class I, (3) patients with 2 or 3 metastases under the age of 50 years, and (4) patients with 2 or 3 metastases and non-small cell lung cancer or any squamous carcinoma. Furthermore, all subsets of patients in the WBRT + SRS group were more likely to have a stable or improved performance status, improved local control and reduced steroid dependence compared to the WBRT alone group. Systemic disease remained the primary cause of death in both groups. Adverse events and the rate of reoperation were comparable in the two groups. Reoperation pathology showed necrosis in all patients in the WBRT + SRS arm and viable tumor in all patients in the WBRT alone arm. Consequently, these two studies provide level 1 evidence that radiosurgery improves local tumor control and is associated with better survival rates in subsets of brain metastases patients.

Three retrospective studies have compared the results of surgical resection to radiosurgery for patients with a single brain metastasis [67–69]. Bindal et al. [67] compared 13 patients having radiosurgery to a matched group of 62 patients having surgical resection. The median survival for the radiosurgery patients was 7.5 months compared to 16.4 months in the microsurgical group ($p = 0.002$). The difference in survival was attributed to progression of the treated tumor in the radiosurgical group, not systemic progression or development of new brain metastatic disease. Muacevic et al. [68] compared 52 patients having microsurgery plus WBRT to 56 patients having only radiosurgery. No difference was noted in survival (53 vs. 43%, $p = 0.19$), local tumor control (75 vs. 83%, $p = 0.49$), or neurologic death rates (37 vs. 39%, $p = 0.80$) 1 year after treatment. Perioperative morbidity and mortality were similar. O'Neill et al. [69] compared 74 patients having microsurgery to 23 patients having radiosurgery. No difference was noted in 1-year survival (62 vs. 56%, p = 0.15); local control was significantly better for the radiosurgery patients (100 vs. 85%, p = 0.02). On the basis of the two larger and more recent papers, patient survival and local tumor control were similar between the microsurgery and radiosurgery groups. However, the potential biases in these papers are substantial and it is difficult to draw any firm conclusions regarding the best treatment for this heterogenous patient population.

Gliomas

Radiosurgery can be used as part of the initial management of patients with high-grade gliomas [64] or as an adjunct for patients with recurrent tumors after completion of conventional therapy [60–63, 65]. Souhami et al. [64] presented the results of the RTOG protocol 93-05. This was an RCT evaluating upfront radiosurgery followed by radiation therapy and BCNU chemotherapy compared to radiation therapy and BCNU chemotherapy for adult patients with supratentorial glioblastoma multiforme less than 4 cm in diameter. Between 1994 and 2000, 203 patients were randomized and 186 were included in the final analysis. No improvement in survival was noted for patients having radiosurgery (median survival, 14.1 vs. 13.7 months, p = 0.53). In addition, patterns of failure and quality of life determinations were similar between the two groups. This trial showed that when used in the upfront management of patients with supratentorial glioblastoma multiforme, radiosurgery did not lead to improved survival or quality of life (level 1 evidence).

Other studies have retrospectively examined the use of radiosurgery typically for recurrent high-grade gliomas after completion of radiation therapy and chemotherapy [60–63, 65]. These studies generally have shown a survival benefit to subgroups of these patients including younger age, better performance status, RTOG class, and histology. However, these studies are subject to significant selection bias and provide rather poor support (level 4 evidence) regarding the role of radiosurgery as an adjunct therapy for recurrent high-grade gliomas.

Vascular Malformations

Arteriovenous Malformations

Arteriovenous malformation (AVM) radiosurgery has been performed for more than 30 years [71–74]. The postradiosurgical obliteration rates, the risk of radiation-related complications, and the chance of a postradiosurgical hemorrhage have each been thoroughly analyzed with the following conclusions. (1) AVM obliteration correlates with the radiation dose delivered to the margin of the malformation [75, 76]. Assuming that the radiation is well targeted, the chance of AVM cure is approximately 70, 80 and 90% for radiation doses of 16, 18 and 20 Gy, respectively. (2) The likelihood of radiation-related complications after AVM radiosurgery relates to some measure of the radiation dose to the surrounding tissue (most commonly used is the 12-Gy volume), and the location of the AVM [77]. (3) Radiosurgery does not increase the bleeding rate of AVMs [78–80].

Several papers have attempted to compare the results of surgical resection and radiosurgery for patients with small- to medium-sized AVMs [81, 82]. In each study, the conclusion was that surgical resection provided higher cure rate with less treatment-associated morbidity. However, closer inspection of the patient characteristics in each group shows that the groups are not directly comparable. For example, approximately one third of patients in most AVM series have AVMs located in the basal ganglia, thalamus, or brainstem, whereas fewer than 10% of patients in microsurgical series have deep AVMs [73]. As a result, the conclusions drawn from these studies are fundamentally flawed and are of little use. Unfortunately, there is little hope that an RCT will ever be performed to compare these two techniques for the reasons previously discussed. Nonetheless, patient outcomes after radiosurgery do compare favorably to historical controls on the natural history of untreated AVMs. So although the best evidence to support AVM radiosurgery is level 4, few clinicians dispute that it plays an important role in the management of AVM patients.

Cavernous Malformations

Cavernous malformation (CM) radiosurgery remains controversial. Problems related to the assessment of the efficacy of CM radiosurgery are 2-fold. First, the incidence and natural history of these lesions remain poorly understood. Second, unlike AVM radiosurgery where obliteration can be confirmed with angiography, CMs often do not change appearance after radiosurgery on MRI and it is the clinical course of the patient that is followed to determine whether radiosurgery has reduced either their risk of bleeding or new neurologic events. Numerous studies have documented a decline in the annual bleeding risk after the first several years [83–87]. However, recent observations that CMs tend to bleed in 'clusters' followed by more quiescent periods creates doubt that radiosurgery has any effect on hemorrhage risk for these patients [88]. Moreover, it has been noted that the risk of radiation-related complications is greater for patients with CMs compared to patients with AVMs, even when lesion size, location, and radiation dose are comparable [83, 86, 87]. Therefore, although the case series data suggest that radiosurgery reduces the hemorrhage rate of CMs (level 4 evidence), the indications for CM radiosurgery remain unclear.

Functional Disorders

When Lars Leksell [2] conceived the idea of radiosurgery, he believed it could be used to noninvasively create precise lesions within the brain to treat functional disorders. In fact, a review of the first 762 cases performed with the Gamma Knife at the Karolinska Institute showed that 63 (8%) were for trigeminal neuralgia. With the advent of MRI, functional radiosurgery has seen a rebirth with it being commonly used to treat trigeminal neuralgia [89–97] and patients with temporal lobe epilepsy [98, 99].

Trigeminal Neuralgia

The reemergence of trigeminal neuralgia radiosurgery can be traced to the publication by Kondziolka et al. [92] in 1996. That study was a multicenter, prospective dose escalation study of patients with idiopathic trigeminal neuralgia. The radiosurgical target was the trigeminal nerve just as it left the brainstem; a single 4-mm isocenter was used to irradiate this structure. At a mean follow-up of 18 months, more than half of the patients became pain-free. The mean time to pain relief was 1 month. Only 3 patients (6%) developed new facial numbness.

Based on the encouraging results of that paper, trigeminal neuralgia radiosurgery has become quite popular and is commonly referred to as the least invasive surgery available for patients with medically unresponsive trigeminal neuralgia. A number of techniques have been used to improve facial pain outcomes including dose escalation [91, 94, 95] and irradiation of a longer segment of the trigeminal nerve [90]. Although the data on higher dose radiosurgery for trigeminal neuralgia has been derived from retrospective studies (level 4 evidence), the published results consistently show that more patients are relieved of their face pain at doses greater than 85 Gy compared to less than 80 Gy. Unfortunately, the incidence of trigeminal dysfunction also appears to increase at higher radiation doses.

The University of Pittsburgh and the Mayo Clinic conducted an RCT comparing one- versus two-shot radiosurgery for trigeminal neuralgia [90]. Eighty-seven patients with idiopathic trigeminal neuralgia were randomized to receive either one-shot (n = 44) or two-shot (n = 43) plans with a maximum dose of 75 Gy. No difference was noted in pain control with a median follow-up of 26 months. The development of facial numbness or paresthesias correlated with the length of irradiated nerve. Although the findings of this paper provide level 1 evidence stating that there was no benefit to patients with the two-shot technique, the majority of recent papers on trigeminal neuralgia radiosurgery have found a clear association between the onset of facial numbness and pain relief after radiosurgery [94, 96]. A larger study in which a longer segment of nerve is irradiated may very well show that this technique provides better facial pain outcomes.

Epilepsy

Over the years an improvement in seizure frequency has often been noted after radiosurgery for patients with epilepsy related to AVMs, CMs, and hypothalamic hamartomas. Regis et al. [99] have studied using radiosurgery to treat patients with drug-resistant mesial temporal lobe epilepsy (MTLE). Sixteen patients had been followed for more than 2 years. Thirteen patients (81%) were seizure free. The median time from radiosurgery to seizure cessation was 10.5 months. Three patients had transient radiation-related complications that required treatment with corticosteroids. Three patients (19%) developed new visual field deficits. This pilot work had prompted a great deal of interest in the use radiosurgery for MTLE. A prospective NIH-funded study is ongoing to more thoroughly investigate the safety and efficacy of MTLE radiosurgery.

References

1 Leksell L: The stereotactic method and radiosurgery of the brain. Acta Chir Scand 1951;107: 316–319.

2 Leksell L: Stereotactic radiosurgery. J Neurol Neurosurg Psychiatry 1983;46:797–803.

3 Pollock BE, Lunsford LD: A call to define stereotactic radiosurgery. Neurosurgery 2004;55: 1371–1373.

4 Sackett DL, Rosenberg WM, Gray JA, Haynes RB, Richardson WS: Evidence based medicine: what it is and what it isn't. BMJ 1996;312:71–72.

5 The periodic health examination. Canadian Task Force on the Periodic Health Examination. Can Med Assoc J 1979;121:1193–1254.

6 Hakim R, Alexander E 3rd, Loeffler JS, Shrieve DC, Wen P, Fallon MP, Steig PE, Black PM: Results of linear accelerator-based radiosurgery for intracranial meningiomas. Neurosurgery 1998;42:446–453.

7 Kondziolka D, Levy EI, Niranjan A, Flickinger JC, Lunsford LD: Long-term outcomes after meningioma radiosurgery: physician and patient perspectives. J Neurosurg 1999;91:44–50.

8 Lee JYK, Niranjan A, McInerney J, Kondziolka D, Flickinger JC, Lunsford LD: Stereotactic radiosurgery providing long-term tumor control of cavernous sinus meningiomas. J Neurosurg 2002;97:65–72.

9 Nicolato A, Foroni R, Alessandrini F, Bricolo A, Gerosa M: Radiosurgical treatment of cavernous sinus meningiomas: experience with 122 treated patients. Neurosurgery 2002;51:1153–1161.

10 Pollock BE, Stafford SL, Utter A, Giannini C, Schreiner SA: Stereotactic radiosurgery provides equivalent tumor control to a Simpson Grade 1 resection for patients with small- to medium-sized meningiomas. Int J Radiat Oncol Biol Phys 2003;55:1000–1005.

11 Shafron DH, Friedman WA, Buatti JM, Bova FJ, Mendenhall WM: Linac radiosurgery for benign meningiomas. Int J Radiat Oncol Biol Phys 1999;43:321–327.

12 Shin M, Kurita H, Sasaki T, Kawamoto S, Tago M, Kawahara N, Morita A, Ueki K, Kirino T: Analysis of treatment outcome after stereotactic radiosurgery for cavernous sinus meningiomas. J Neurosurg 2001;95:435–439.

13 Stafford SL, Pollock BE, Foote RL, Gorman DA, Schomberg PJ, Leavitt JA: Meningioma radiosurgery: tumor control, outcomes, and complications in 190 consecutive patients. Neurosurgery 2001;49:1029–1038.

14 Flickinger JC, Kondziolka D, Niranjan A, Lunsford LD: Results of acoustic neuroma radiosurgery: an analysis of 5 years' experience using current methods. J Neurosurg 2001;94:1–6.
15 Foote KD, Freidman WA, Buatti JM, Meeks SL, Bova FJ, Kubilis PS: Analysis of risk factors associated with radiosurgery for vestibular schwannoma. J Neurosurg 2001;95:440–449.
16 Iwai Y, Yamanaka K, Shiotani M, Uyama T: Radiosurgery for acoustic neuromas: results of low-dose treatment. Neurosurgery 2003;53:282–287.
17 Karpinos M, The BS, Zeck O, Carpenter LS, Phan C, Mai W, Lu HH, Chiu JK, Butler EB, Gormley WB, Woo SY: Treatment of acoustic neuroma: stereotactic radiosurgery vs. microsurgery. Int J Radiat Oncol Biol Phys 2002;54:1410–1421.
18 Kondziolka D, Lunsford LD, McLaughlin MR, Flickinger JC: Long-term outcomes after radiosurgery for acoustic neuromas. N Engl J Med 1998;339:1426–1433.
19 Petit JH, Hudes RS, Chen TT, Eisenberg HM, Simard JM, Chin LS: Reduced-dose radiosurgery for vestibular schwannomas. Neurosurgery 2001;49:1299–1306.
20 Pollock BE, Lunsford LD, Kondziolka D, Flickinger JC, Bissonette DJ, Kelsey SF, Jannetta PJ: Outcome analysis of acoustic neuroma management: a comparison of microsurgery and stereotactic radiosurgery. Neurosurgery 1995;36:215–223.
21 Prasad D, Steiner M, Steiner L: Gamma surgery for vestibular schwannoma. J Neurosurg 2000;92: 745–759.
22 Regis J, Pellet W, Delsanti C, Dufour H, Roche PH, Thomassin JM, Zanaret M, Peragut JC: Functional outcome after gamma knife surgery or microsurgery for vestibular schwannomas. J Neurosurg 2002;97:1091–1100.
23 Van Roijen L, Nijs HGT, Avezaat CJJ, Karlsson B, Lindquist C, Pauw KH, Rutten FFH: Costs and effects of microsurgery versus radiosurgery in treating acoustic neuromas. Acta Neurochir (Wien) 1997;139:942–948.
24 Huang CF, Kondziolka D, Flickinger JC, Lunsford LD: Stereotactic radiosurgery for trigeminal schwannomas. Neurosurgery 1999;45:11–16.
25 Mabanta SR, Buatti JM, Friedman WA, Meeks SL, Mendenhall WM, Bova FJ: Linear accelerator radiosurgery for nonacoustic schwannomas. Int J Radiat Oncol Biol Phys 1999;43:545–548.
26 Muthukumar N, Kondziolka D, Lunsford LD, Flickinger JC: Stereotactic radiosurgery for jugular foramen schwannomas. Surg Neurol 1999;52:172–179.
27 Pollock BE, Foote RL, Stafford SL: Stereotactic radiosurgery: the preferred management for patients with non-vestibular schwannomas? Int J Radiat Oncol Biol Phys 2002;52:1002–1007.
28 Ikeda H, Jokura H, Yoshimoto T: Transsphenoidal surgery and adjuvant gamma knife treatment for growth hormone-secreting pituitary adenoma. J Neurosurg 2001;95:285–291.
29 Landolt AM, Haller D, Lomax N, Scheib S, Schubiger O, Siegfreid T, Wellis G: Stereotactic radiosurgery for recurrent surgically treated acromegaly: comparison with fractionated radiotherapy. J Neurosurg 1998;88:1002–1008.
30 Landolt AM, Haller D, Lomax N, Scheib S, Schubiger O, Siegfreid T, Wellis G: Octreotide may act as a radioprotective agent in acromegaly. J Clin Endocrinol Metab 2000;85:1287–1289.
31 Landolt AM, Lomax N: Gamma knife radiosurgery for prolactinomas. J Neurosurg 2000;93(suppl 3): 14–18.
32 Pollock BE, Nippoldt TB, Stafford SL, Foote RL, Abboud CF: Results of stereotactic radiosurgery for patients with hormone producing pituitary adenomas: factors associated with endocrine normalization. J Neurosurg 2002;97:525–530.
33 Pollock BE, Young WF Jr: Stereotactic radiosurgery for patients with ACTH-producing pituitary adenomas after prior adrenalectomy. Int J Radiat Oncol Biol Phys 2002;54:839–841.
34 Pollock BE, Carpenter PC: Stereotactic radiosurgery as an alternative to fractionated radiation therapy for patients with recurrent or residual nonfunctioning pituitary adenomas. Neurosurgery 2003;53:1086–1094.
35 Sheehan JM, Vance ML, Sheehan JP, Ellegala DB, Laws ER Jr: Radiosurgery for Cushing's disease after failed transsphenoidal surgery. J Neurosurg 2000;93:738–742.
36 Sheehan JP, Kondziolka D, Flickinger JC, Lunsford LD: Radiosurgery for residual or recurrent nonfunctioning pituitary adenoma. J Neurosurg 2002;97(suppl 5):408–414.
37 Linskey ME: Stereotactic radiosurgery versus stereotactic radiotherapy for patients with vestibular schwannomas: a Leksell Gamma Knife Society 2000 debate. J Neurosurg 2000;93(suppl 3):90–95.

38 Nikolopoulos TP, O'Donoghue GM: Acoustic neuroma management: an evidence-based medicine approach. Otol Neurotol 2002;23:534–541.
39 Kaylie DM, McMenomey SO: Microsurgery vs. gamma knife radiosurgery for the treatment of vestibular schwannomas. Arch Otolarynolgol Head Neck Surg 2003;129:903–906.
40 Pollock BE, Lunsford LD, Noren G: Vestibular schwannoma management in the next century: a radiosurgical perspective. Neurosurgery 1998;43:475–483.
41 Sekhar LN, Gormley WB, Wright DC: The best treatment for vestibular schwannoma (acoustic neuroma): microsurgery or radiosurgery? Am J Otol 1996;17:676–682.
42 Andrews DW, Suarez O, Goldman HW, Downes MB, Bednarz G, Corn BW, Werner-Wasik M, Rosenstock J, Curran WJ Jr: Stereotactic radiosurgery and fractionated stereotactic radiotherapy for the treatment of acoustic schwannomas: comparative observations of 125 patients treated at one institution. Int J Radiat Oncol Biol Phys 2001;50:1265–1278.
43 Meijer OW, Vandertop WP, Baayen JC, Slotman BJ: Single-fraction vs. fractionated linac-based stereotactic radiosurgery for vestibular schwannoma: a single-institution study. Int J Radiat Oncol Biol Phys 2003;56:1390–1396.
44 Alexander E 3rd, Moriarty TM, Davis RB, Wen PY, Fine HA, Black PMcL, Kooy HM, Loeffler JS: Stereotactic radiosurgery for the definitive, noninvasive treatment of brain metastases. J Natl Cancer Inst 1995;87:34–40.
45 Auchter RM, Lamond JP, Alexander E 3rd, Buatti JM, Chappell R, Friedman WA, Knisella TJ, Levin AB, Noyes WR, Schultz CJ, Loeffler JS, Mehta MP: A multiinstitutional outcome and prognostic factor analysis of radiosurgery for resectable single brain metastasis. Int J Radiat Oncol Biol Phys 1996;35:27–35.
46 Brown PD, Brown CA, Pollock BE, Gorman DA, Foote RL: Stereotactic radiosurgery for patients with radioresistant brain metastases. Neurosurgery 2002;51:656–667.
47 Buatti JM, Friedman WA, Bova FJ, Mendenhall WM: Treatment selection factors for stereotactic radiosurgery of intracranial metastases. Int J Radiat Oncol Biol Phys 1995;32:1161–1166.
48 Flickinger JC, Kondziolka D, Lunsford LD, Coffey RJ, Goodman ML, Shaw EG, Hudgins WR, Weiner R, Harsh GR, Sneed PK, Larson DA: A multi-institutional experience with stereotactic radiosurgery for solitary brain metastasis. Int J Radiat Oncol Biol Phys 1994;28:797–802.
49 Joseph J, Adler JR, Cox RS, Hancock SL: Linear accelerator-based stereotactic radiosurgery for brain metastases: the influence of number of lesions on survival. J Clin Oncol 1996;14: 1085–1092.
50 Kondziolka D, Patel A, Lunsford LD, Kassam A, Flickinger JC: Stereotactic radiosurgery plus whole brain radiotherapy versus radiotherapy alone for patients with multiple brain metastases. Int J Radiat Oncol Biol Phys 1999;45:427–434.
51 Lavine SD, Petrovich Z, Cohen-Gadol AA, Marsi LS, Morton DL, O'Day SJ, Essner R, Zelman V, Yu C, Luxton G, Apuzzo MLJ: Gamma knife radiosurgery for metastatic melanoma: an analysis of survival, outcome, and complications. Neurosurgery 1999;44:59–66.
52 Matsuo T, Shibata S, Yasunga A, Iwanaga M, Mori K, Shimizu T, Hayashi N, Ochi M, Hayashi K: Dose optimization and indications of Linac radiosurgery for brain metastases. Int J Radiat Oncol Biol Phys 1999;45:931–939.
53 Mori Y, Kondziolka D, Lunsford LD, Logan T, Flickinger JC: Stereotactic radiosurgery for brain metastases from renal cell carcinoma. Cancer 1998;83:344–353.
54 Nussbaum ES, Djalilian HR, Cho KH, Hall WA: Brain metastases: histology, multiplicity, surgery and survival. Cancer 1996;78:1781–1788.
55 Pirzkall A, Debrus J, Lohr F, Fuss M, Rhein B, Engenhart-Cabillic R, Wannenmacher M: Radiosurgery alone or in conjunction with whole-brain radiotherapy for brain metastases. J Clin Oncol 1998;16:3563–3569.
56 Pollock BE, Brown PD, Foote RL, Stafford SL, Schomberg PJ: Properly selected patients with multiple brain metastases may benefit from aggressive treatment of their intracranial disease. J Neurooncol 2003;61:73–80.
57 Schoeggl A, Kitz K, Ertel A, Reddy M, Bavinski G, Schneider B: Prognostic factor analysis for multiple brain metastases after gamma knife radiosurgery: results in 97 patients. J Neurooncol 1999;42:169–175.

58 Sneed PK, Lamborn KR, Forstner JM, McDermott MW, Chang S, Park E, Gutin PH, Phillips TL, Wara WM, Larson DA: Radiosurgery for brain metastases: is whole brain radiotherapy necessary. Int J Radiat Oncol Biol Phys 1999;43:549–558.
59 Weltman E, Salvajoli JV, Brandt RA, Hanriot RM, Prisco FE, Cruz JC, De Oliveria SR, Wajsbrot DB: Radiosurgery for brain metastases: a score index for predicting prognosis. Int J Radiat Oncol Biol Phys 2000;46:1155–1161.
60 Graves EE, Nelson SJ, Vigneron DB, Chin C, Verhay L, McDermott M, Larson D, Sneed PK, Chang S, Prados MD, Lamborn K, Dillon WP: A preliminary study on the prognostic value of proton magnetic resonance spectroscopic imaging in gamma knife radiosurgery of recurrent malignant gliomas. Neurosurgery 2000;46:319–326.
61 Kondziolka D, Flickinger JC, Bissonette DJ, Bozik M, Lunsford LD: Survival benefit of stereotactic radiosurgery for patients with malignant glial neoplasms. Neurosurgery 1997;41:776–783.
62 Nwokedi EC, DiBiase SJ, Jabbour S, Herman J, Amin P, Chin LS: Gamma knife stereotactic radiosurgery for patients with glioblastoma multiforme. Neurosurgery 2002;50:41–46.
63 Shrieve DC, Alexander E 3rd, Black PM, Wen PY, Fine HA, Kooy HM, Loeffler JS: Treatment of patients with primary glioblastoma multiforme with standard postoperative radiotherapy and radiosurgical boost: prognostic factors and long-term outcome. J Neurosurg 1999;90:72–77.
64 Souhami L, Seiferheld W, Brachman D, Podgorsak EB, Werner-Wasik M, Lustig R, Schultz CJ, Sause W, Okunieff P, Buckner J, Zamorano L, Mehta MP, Curran WJ Jr: Randomized comparison of stereotactic radiosurgery followed by conventional radiotherapy with carmustine to conventional radiotherapy with carmustine for patients with glioblastoma multiforme: report of the Radiation Therapy Oncology Group 93-05 protocol. Int J Radiat Oncol Biol Phys 2004:60:853–860.
65 Shaw EG, Scott C, Souhami L, Dinapoli R, Kline R, Loeffler J, Farnan N: Single dose radiosurgical treatment of recurrent previously irradiated primary tumors and brain metastases: final report of RTOG protocol 90-05. Int J Radiat Oncol Biol Phys 2000;47:291–298.
66 Shaw EG: Radiotherapeutic management of multiple brain metastases: '3000 in 10' whole brain radiation is no longer a 'no brainer'. Int J Radiat Oncol Biol Phys 1999;45:253–254.
67 Bindal AK, Bindal RK, Hess KR, Shiu A, Hassenbusch SJ, Shi WM, Sawaya R: Surgery versus radiosurgery in the treatment of brain metastasis. J Neurosurg 1996;84:748–754.
68 Muacevic A, Kreth FW, Horstmann GA, Schmid-Elsaesser R, Wowra B, Steiger HJ, Reulen HJ: Surgery and radiotherapy compared to gamma knife radiosurgery in the treatment of solitary cerebral metastases of small diameter. J Neurosurg 1999;91:35–43.
69 O'Neill BP, Iturria NJ, Link MJ, Pollock BE, Ballman KV, O'Fallon JR: A comparison of surgical resection and stereotactic radiosurgery in the treatment of solitary brain metastases. Int J Radiat Oncol Biol Phys 2003;55:1169–1176.
70 Andrews DW, Scott CB, Sperduto PW, Flanders AE, Gaspar LE, Schell MC, Werner-Wasik M, Demas W, Ryu J, Bahary J, Souhami L, Rotman M, Mehta MP, Curran WJ Jr: Whole brain radiation therapy with or without stereotactic radiosurgery boost for patients with one to three brain metastases: phase III results of the RTOG 9508 randomised trial. Lancet 2004;363:1665–1672.
71 Friedman WA, Bova FJ, Bollampally S, Bradshaw P: Analysis of factors predictive of success or complications in arteriovenous malformation radiosurgery. Neurosurgery 2003;52:296–308.
72 Kjellberg RN, Hanamura T, Davis KR, Lyons SL, Adams RD: Bragg-peak proton-beam therapy for arteriovenous malformations. N Engl J Med 1983;309:269–274.
73 Pollock BE, Flickinger JC: A proposed radiosurgery-based grading system for arteriovenous malformations. J Neurosurg 2002;96:79–85.
74 Pollock BE, Gorman DA, Coffey RJ: Patient outcomes after arteriovenous malformation radiosurgical management: results based on a 5- to 14-year follow-up study. Neurosurgery 2003;52:1291–1297.
75 Flickinger JC, Pollock BE, Kondziolka D, Lunsford LD: A dose-response analysis of arteriovenous malformation obliteration by radiosurgery. Int J Radiat Onc Biol Phys 1996;36:873–879.
76 Karlsson B, Lindquist C, Steiner L: Prediction of obliteration after gamma knife surgery for cerebral arteriovenous malformations. Neurosurgery 1997;40:425–431.
77 Flickinger JC, Kondziolka D, Lunsford LD, Liscak R, Phuong LK, Pollock BE: Development of a model to predict permanent symptomatic post-radiosurgery injury for arteriovenous malformation patients. Int J Radiat Oncol Biol Phys 2000;46:1143–1148.

78 Friedman WA, Blatt DL, Bova FJ, Buatti JM, Mendenhall WM, Kubilis PS: The risk of hemorrhage after radiosurgery for arteriovenous malformations. J Neurosurg 1996;84:912–919.
79 Karlsson B, Lax I, Söderman M: Risk of hemorrhage during the 2-year latency period following gamma knife radiosurgery for arteriovenous malformations. Int J Radiat Oncol Biol Phys 2001; 49:1045–1051.
80 Pollock BE, Flickinger JC, Lunsford LD, Bissonette DJ, Kondziolka D: Hemorrhage risk after stereotactic radiosurgery of cerebral arteriovenous malformations. Neurosurgery 1996;38: 652–661.
81 Pikus HJ, Beach ML, Harbaugh RE: Microsurgical treatment of arteriovenous malformations: analysis and comparison with stereotactic radiosurgery. J Neurosurg 1998;88:641–646.
82 Porter PJ, Shin AY, Detsky AS, Lefaive L, Wallace MC: Surgery versus stereotactic radiosurgery for small, operable cerebral arteriovenous malformations: a clinical and cost comparison. Neurosurgery 1997;41:757–766.
83 Amin-Hanjabi S, Ogilvy CS, Candia GJ, Lyons S, Chapman PH: Stereotactic radiosurgery for cavernous malformations: Kjellberg's experience with proton beam therapy in 98 cases at the Harvard cyclotron. Neurosurgery 1998;42:1229–1238.
84 Chang SD, Levy RP, Adler JR Jr, Martin DP, Krakovitz PR, Steinberg GK: Stereotactic radiosurgery of angiographically occult vascular malformations: 14-year experience. Neurosurgery 1998;43:213–221.
85 Hasegawa T, McInerney J, Kondziolka D, Lee JY, Flickinger JC, Lunsford LD: Long-term results after stereotactic radiosurgery for patients with cavernous malformations. Neurosurgery 2002;50:1190–1197.
86 Karlsson B, Kihlström L, Lindquist C, Ericson K, Steiner L: Radiosurgery for cavernous malformations. J Neurosurg 1998;88:293–297.
87 Pollock BE, Garces YI, Stafford SL, Foote RL, Schomberg PJ, Link ML: Stereotactic radiosurgery of cavernous malformations. J Neurosurg 2000;93:987–991.
88 Barker FG 2nd, Amin-Hanjabi S, Butler WE, Lyons S, Ojemann RG, Chapman PH, Ogilvy CS: Temporal clustering of hemorrhages from untreated cavernous malformations of the central nervous system. Neurosurgery 2001;49:15–25.
89 Brisman R: Gamma knife radiosurgery with a dose of 75 to 76.8 Gy for trigeminal neuralgia. J Neurosurg 2004;100:848–854.
90 Flickinger JC, Pollock BE, Kondziolka D, Phuong LK, Foote RL, Stafford SL, Lunsford LD: What length should be irradiated? A randomized blinded study of radiosurgery to different lengths of trigeminal nerve for trigeminal neuralgia. Int J Radiat Oncol Biol Phys 2001;51:449–454.
91 Goss BW, Frighetto L, DeSalles AAF, Smith Z, Solberg T, Selch M: Linear accelerator radiosurgery using 90 Gy for essential trigeminal neuralgia: results and dose volume histogram analysis. Neurosurgery 2003;53:823–830.
92 Kondziolka D, Lunsford LD, Flickinger JC, Young RF, Vermeulen S, Duma CM, Jacques DB, Rand RW, Regis J, Peragut JC, Manera L, Epstein MH, Lindquist C: Stereotactic radiosurgery for trigeminal neuralgia: a multiinstutional study using the gamma unit. J Neurosurg 1996;84: 940–945.
93 Maesawa S, Salame C, Flickinger JC, Pirris S, Kondziolka D, Lunsford LD: Clinical outcomes after stereotactic radiosurgery for idiopathic trigeminal neuralgia. J Neurosurg 2001;94:14–20.
94 Massager N, Lorenzoni J, Devriendt D, Desmedt F, Brotchi J, Levivier M: Gamma knife surgery for idiopathic trigeminal neuralgia performed using a far-anterior cisternal target and a high dose of radiation. J Neurosurg 2004;100:597–605.
95 Pollock BE, Phuong LK, Foote RL, Stafford SL, Gorman DA: High-dose trigeminal neuralgia radiosurgery associated with increased risk of trigeminal dysfunction. Neurosurgery 2001;49: 58–64.
96 Pollock BE, Phuong LK, Gorman DA, Foote RL, Stafford SL, Schomberg PJ: Stereotactic radiosurgery for idiopathic trigeminal neuralgia. J Neurosurg 2002;97:347–353.
97 Smith ZA, DeSalles AAF, Frighetto L, Goss B, Lee SP, Selch M, Wallace RE, Cabatan-Awang C, Solberg T: Dedicated linear accelerator radiosurgery for the treatment of trigeminal neuralgia. J Neurosurg 2003;99:511–516.

98 Kondziolka D: Functional radiosurgery. Neurosurgery 1999;44:12–22.
99 Regis J, Bartolomei F, Rey M, Hayashi M, Chauvel P, Peragut JC: Gamma knife surgery for mesial temporal lobe epilepsy. J Neurosurg 2000;93(suppl 3):141–146.

Bruce E. Pollock, MD
Department of Neurological Surgery, Mayo Clinic
200 First Street SW
Rochester, MN 55905 (USA)
Tel. +1 507 284 5317, Fax +1 507 284 5206, E-Mail pollock.bruce@mayo.edu

Pollock BE (ed): Guiding Neurosurgery by Evidence.
Prog Neurol Surg. Basel, Karger, 2006, vol 19, pp 171–196

Evidenced-Based Guidelines for Traumatic Brain Injuries

Donald W. Marion

Fusion Medical Education, LLC, Wakefield, Mass., USA

Abstract

An enormous amount of clinical and basic science brain injury research has been undertaken during the last several decades in an effort to improve outcomes following severe traumatic brain injury, but to date there still are no new therapies that have been clearly shown to be beneficial. There is, however, increasing evidence to suggest that evidence-based, protocol-driven, acute care can lead to improved outcomes. Evidence based guidelines for the medical and surgical management of severe brain injury, and for penetrating and pediatric brain injury, as well as for the pre-hospital management of brain injury, have all been published. In this chapter the conclusions of those guidelines is reviewed. In addition, the studies that demonstrate improved outcomes as a result of implementation of the guidelines are summarized.

Nearly a century ago surgeons discovered that evacuation of posttraumatic hematomas could, in some cases at least, lead to survival and even good outcomes. But by the 1950s it also was recognized that many of those with severe traumatic brain injury (TBI) died of intracranial hypertension due to brain swelling. Since that time there has been extensive research aimed at refining intracranial pressure (ICP) monitoring techniques, defining the physiologic and molecular causes of posttraumatic brain swelling, and identifying therapies that ameliorate brain swelling and lead to improved outcomes. Much of the research conducted during the past 20 years has focused on a relatively small number of molecular mechanisms identified in rodent models of TBI to be critical intermediates of secondary brain injury. Drugs were developed that could effectively block some of these mechanisms of secondary injury (in laboratory models), and those drugs were tested in large-scale multicenter clinical trials. To date numerous clinical trials have been completed but none have shown improved outcomes as a result of the novel treatment.

Because of the lack of therapies proven to reduce brain swelling, many neurosurgeons and other clinicians involved in the care of TBI patients adopted therapeutic biases based on personal experience, incomplete literature reviews, or the views of their mentors. This led to a tremendous degree of variability of practice throughout the US. A survey of US trauma centers conducted by the Brain Trauma Foundation in 1991 found that there was significant disagreement about the need for ICP monitoring, role of steroids, and role of barbiturates for patients with severe TBI [1]. As a result, there was considerable controversy and confusion within hospital intensive care units because of inconsistent treatment of the TBI patients depending on who was responsible for their care during a particular day or week.

The rationale for the development and implementation of evidence-based guidelines in TBI care is 2-fold: first, that there are 'best practices', and second, that consistent care within and among hospitals treating TBI patients will lead to improved outcomes. The strength of guidelines in part relies on the availability of good quality studies that document improved outcomes with the use of one particular treatment compared to the management of the patient without that treatment, or with the use of an alternative treatment. It is generally accepted that such studies should be prospective randomized controlled clinical trials of large numbers of patients. But even in the absence of such 'class I' studies, a group of lesser quality studies that are consistent in their findings can provide support for guidelines. While such studies may not be used to support a standard of care for a particular treatment recommendation, they can be used to craft guidelines or options. In some cases, support for best practices must rely on indirect evidence, or intuitive science. For example, intracranial hypertension is known to be an important proximate cause for neurologic morbidity and mortality following TBI. It is logical to conclude that treatment of intracranial hypertension cannot be effectively accomplished unless the clinician knows what the ICP is. Most clinicians consider the reduction of ICP an important indicator of the effectiveness of treatment. In addition, it is believed that despite a lack of prospective randomized clinical trials in support of specific treatment recommendations, the creation of guidelines supported by the best available literature is justified because they promote consistent acute care of TBI patients. Consistent protocol-driven care helps to establish a team approach, eliminates confusion, and is thereby likely to lead to improved outcomes.

History of Contemporary TBI Guideline Development

During the early 1990s a small group of neurosurgeons who were interested in neurotrauma agreed that there was a need to standardize care of patients with severe TBI according to best practice guidelines. They believed that the wide variability of care provided by neurosurgeons throughout the US was likely responsible for preventable death and disability in a significant proportion of TBI patients. At the same time, the Agency for Health Care Policy and Research (AHCPR), Department of Health and Human Services, had made the same conclusion for all of medicine and was promoting the development of evidence-based guidelines for all medical specialties [2]. The neurosurgeons embraced the methodology for development of evidence-based guidelines developed by AHCPR and, with the financial support of the Brain Trauma Foundation, produced the Guidelines for the Management of Severe Head Injury. Using the AHCPR methodology, 11 neurosurgeons with an interest in TBI selected 13 topics considered most important for the care of TBI patients. Each neurosurgeon was assigned a topic and proceeded with a thorough literature search to identify all related peer-reviewed journal articles (primarily English language) that were published over the last 40 years. The studies were then categorized as class I (prospective randomized controlled clinical trials), class II (nonrandomized cohort studies, randomized controlled clinical trials with significant design flaws, or case-controlled studies), or class III (expert opinion, case reports, most retrospective studies). Recommendations were formulated for each topic, and considered as 'standards' if supported by one or more class I studies, 'guidelines' if supported by two or more class II studies, or 'options' if supported only by class III studies. A draft document was produced with a separate chapter for each topic, and the document was widely circulated to all medical specialties and organizations with a stake in the care of TBI patients for their input. A final document was produced after incorporating the suggestions of these organizations. The document was endorsed by the American Association of Neurological Surgeons and disseminated free of charge to all practicing neurosurgeons in North America in 1995 [3]. Neurosurgeons, as well as trauma surgeons and critical care intensivists, quickly adopted the guidelines and, according to subsequent surveys, often changed their practice to conform to these recommendations. As per an agreement with the American Association of Neurological Surgeons the Guidelines were updated in 2000, and a section was added on prognostic indicators following severe TBI [4].

As a result of the success of this document there was renewed interest in developing evidence-based guidelines for TBI issues not specifically addressed in the Guidelines for the Management of Severe Head Injuries. To date, guidelines have also been completed for the prehospital management of TBI patients [5], the management of penetrating brain injuries [6], and the management of pediatric head injuries [7]. Guidelines for the surgical management of TBI are in press. The authors of these more recent guidelines have faithfully followed the same methodology as was used for development of the original head injury guidelines.

In this chapter the Guidelines for the Management of Severe Traumatic Brain Injury and Early Indicators of Prognosis in Severe Traumatic Brain Injury, Pre-Hospital Management of Traumatic Brain Injury, Management and Prognosis of Penetrating Brain Injury, Guidelines for the Acute Management of Severe Traumatic Brain Injury in Infants, Children, and Adolescents, and the Surgical Management of TBI are summarized by presenting the recommendations of each document. The authors of the guidelines are listed in alphabetical order (by agreement of the authors) in the sections describing the recommendations of each of the Guidelines documents. Several problems with guidelines' development are then addressed, followed by a summary of several recent studies that have looked at the impact of the guidelines on change in practice, and on outcomes following severe TBI. Numerous guidelines for the management of *mild* TBI have appeared over the last 10 years, including sports-related concussion guidelines. These guidelines are not covered in this chapter because most are not truly evidence-based.

Guidelines for the Management of Severe Head Injury, and Early Indicators of Prognosis in Severe Traumatic Brain Injury

This document is the updated version of the original Guidelines document, and was published in 2000 in a special edition of the *Journal of Neurotrauma* [4]. The authors of the section on the Management of Severe Head Injury are M. Ross Bullock, Randall M. Chesnut, Guy L. Clifton, Jamshid Ghajar, Donald W. Marion, Raj K. Narayan, David W. Newell, Lawrence H. Pitts, Michael J. Rosner, Beverly C. Walters, and Jack E. Wilberger (table 1). For the Section on Early Indicators of Prognosis in Severe Traumatic Brain Injury, the authors are Randall M. Chesnut, Jamshid Ghajar, Andrew I.R. Maas, Donald W. Marion, Franco Servadei, Graham M. Teasdale, Andreas Unterberg, Hans von Holst, and Beverly C. Walters (table 2). The document includes an extensive section on the methodology for evidence-based guideline development. Each subsequent chapter covers a specific topic relevant to the acute care of patients with severe TBI. The chapters are written in the same format, with a section on recommendations followed by sections entitled overview, process, scientific foundation, summary, key issues for future investigation, evidentiary tables, and a complete bibliography of studies cited. The recommendations section

Table 1. Guidelines for the Management of Severe Traumatic Brain Injury (adults) [4]

	Standard	Guideline	Option
Trauma systems	None	All regions should have an organized trauma care system	Neurosurgeons should have an organized and responsive system of care for patients with neurotrauma. They should initiate neurotrauma care planning including prehospital management and triage, direct trauma center transport, maintain appropriate call schedules, review trauma care records for quality improvement, and participate in trauma education programs. Trauma facilities treating patients with severe or moderate head injury must have a neurosurgery service, an in-house trauma surgeon, a neurosurgeon promptly available, and a continuously staffed and available operating room, intensive care unit, and laboratory with proper equipment for treating neurotrauma patients. A CT scanner must be immediately available at all times. In rural communities without a neurosurgeon, a properly trained general surgeon may perform emergency life-saving trauma craniotomies
Initial management	None	None	The first priority is complete and rapid physiologic resuscitation. No specific treatment should be directed at intracranial hypertension in the absence of signs of transtentorial herniation or progressive neurologic deterioration not attributable to extracranial explanations. When signs of herniation or progressive deterioration not attributable to extracranial causes are present, the physician should assume that intracranial hypertension exists and treat it aggressively.

Table 1. (continued)

	Standard	Guideline	Option
			Sedation and neuromuscular blockade can be useful in optimizing transport of the patient
Resuscitation of blood pressure and oxygenation	None	Hypotension or hypoxia must be monitored and scrupulously avoided, if possible, or corrected immediately	The mean arterial blood pressure should be maintained above 90 mm Hg through the infusion of fluids throughout the patient's course to attempt to maintain CPP greater than 60 mm Hg. Patients with a GCS <9, who are unable to maintain their airway or who remain hypoxemic despite supplemental O_2, require that their airway be secured, preferably by endotracheal intubation
Indications for ICP monitoring	None	ICP monitoring is appropriate in patients with severe TBI (postresuscitation GCS 3–8) with an abnormal admission CT scan. It also is appropriate in such patients with a normal CT scan if at least 2 of the following exist: age >40 years, motor posturing, or hypotension. ICP monitoring is not routinely indicated in patients with mild or moderate TBI. However, a physician may choose to monitor in certain such patients with mass lesions	

Table 1. (continued)

	Standard	Guideline	Option
ICP treatment threshold	None	ICP treatment should be initiated at an upper threshold of 20–25 mmHg	Interpretation and treatment of ICP based on any threshold should be corroborated by frequent clinical examination and CPP data
CPP	None	CPP should be maintained at a minimum of 60 mm Hg. In the absence of cerebral ischemia, aggressive attempts to maintain a CPP above 70 mm Hg with fluids and pressors should be avoided because the risk of adult respiratory distress syndrome	None
Hyperventilation	In the absence of increased ICP, chronic prolonged hyperventilation therapy should be avoided	Prophylactic hyperventilation therapy during the first 24 h after injury should be avoided because it can compromise cerebral perfusion during a time when CBF is reduced	Hyperventilation therapy may be necessary for brief periods when there is acute neurologic deterioration, or for longer periods if there is intracranial hypertension refractory to sedation, paralysis, CSF drainage, or osmotic diuretics. Jugular venous oxygen saturation, $AVdO_2$, brain tissue oxygen monitoring, or CBF monitoring may help to identify cerebral ischemia if hyperventilation therapy is necessary
Mannitol	None	Mannitol is effective for control of raised ICP. Effective doses range from 0.25 to 1 g/kg	The indications for the use of mannitol prior to ICP monitoring are signs of transtentorial herniation or progressive neurologic deterioration not attributable to extracranial explanations. However, hypovolemia should be avoided by fluid replacement. Serum osmolarity should be kept below 320 mosm because of concern for renal failure. Euvolemia should be maintained by adequate fluid replacement. A Foley catheter is essential. Intermittent boluses may be more effective than continuous infusion

Table 1. (continued)

	Standard	Guideline	Option
Barbiturates	None	High-dose barbiturate therapy may be considered in hemodynamically stable, salvageable patients with intracranial hypertension refractory to maximal medical and surgical treatment	None
Steroids	The use of steroids is not recommended for improving outcome or reducing ICP	None	None
Nutrition	None	Replace 140% of resting metabolic expenditure in nonparalyzed patients and 100% of resting metabolic expenditure in paralyzed patients using enteral or parenteral formulas containing at least 15% of calories as protein by the 7th day after injury	The preferable option is use of jejunal feeding by gastrojejunostomy due to ease of use and avoidance of gastric intolerance
Antiseizure prophylaxis	Prophylactic use of phenytoin, carbamazepine, phenobarbital or valproate is not recommended for preventing late posttraumatic seizures	None	Anticonvulsants may be used to prevent early posttraumatic seizures in patients at high risk for seizures following head injury. Phenytoin and carbamazepine have been demonstrated to be effective in preventing early posttraumatic seizures. However, the available evidence does not indicate that prevention of early posttraumatic seizures improves outcome following head injury

CBF = Cerebral blood flow; CPP = cerebral perfusion pressure.

Table 2. Early Prognostic Indicators following Severe Traumatic Brain Injury [4]

	Features of the parameter supported by class I and strong class II evidence and have at least a 70% positive predictive value for poor outcome
GCS	There is an increasing probability of poor outcome with a decreasing GCS in a continuous, stepwise manner
Age	There is an increasing probability of poor outcome with increasing age in a stepwise manner
Pupillary diameter and light reflex	Bilaterally absent pupillary light reflexes
Hypotension	A systolic blood pressure less than 90 mm Hg was found to have a 67% positive predictive value for poor outcome and, when combined with hypoxia, a 79% positive predictive value for poor outcome
CT scan features	(1) Presence of abnormalities on initial CT (2) CT classification (3) Compressed or absent basal cisterns (4) Traumatic subarachnoid hemorrhage, including blood in the basal cisterns or extensive traumatic subarachnoid hemorrhage

succinctly lists the standards, guidelines and options as supported by the available literature.

In addition to these 'treatment' guidelines, a chapter was devoted to ICP monitoring technology, and the following recommendation derived: 'In the current state of technology the ventricular catheter connected to an external strain gauge is the most accurate, low-cost, and reliable method of monitoring ICP. It also allows therapeutic CSF drainage. ICP transduction via fiberoptic or strain gauge devices placed in ventricular catheters provide similar benefits, but at a higher cost. Parenchymal ICP monitoring with fiberoptic or strain gauge catheter tip transduction is similar to ventricular ICP monitoring but has the potential for measurement drift. Subarachnoid, subdural, and epidural monitors are currently less accurate.'

The most recent edition of the Guidelines for the Management of Severe Traumatic Brain Injury also included a section on Early Prognostic Indicators following Severe TBI (table 2). For this section, several clinical characteristics of severe TBI were selected as most important for determining prognosis. In each case literature searches were conducted and relevant articles reviewed to determine if the prognostic indicator had at least a 70% positive predictive value for determining poor outcome. If so, the details regarding use of the prognostic indicator that were most closely associated with prognosis were defined.

In addition to information about the positive predictive values for each of these characteristics, the prognosis guidelines included recommendations for how the parameter should be measured, when it should be measured, and who should measure it. The section on CT scan features includes subsections detailing the prognostic value of specific CT findings, focusing on the status of the basal cisterns, traumatic subarachnoid hemorrhage, midline shift, and intracranial lesions.

Prehospital Management of Traumatic Brain Injury

The Guidelines for Prehospital Management of Traumatic Brain Injury were published in 2002 in the *Journal of Neurotrauma* by the Brain Trauma Foundation, with financial assistance provided by a grant from the National Highway Traffic Safety Administration [5] (table 3). The authors of the document were Edward J. Gabriel, Jamshid Ghajar, Andrew Jagoda, Peter T. Pons, Thomas Scalea, and Beverly C. Walters. Their specialties included emergency medical technologist, emergency medicine, trauma surgery, and neurosurgery. The authors of these guidelines focused on recommendations for prehospital assessment of the TBI patient and transport decisions, as well as treatment recommendations. However, the assessment category presented a challenge in terms of formulating meaningful recommendations. For example, the relevant question regarding clinical assessment measures is whether or not the measure is reliable, while the relevant question for a treatment is whether or not it is efficacious. A methodology had to be developed to weigh the significance of the literature supporting clinical assessment measures. This methodology, which is thoroughly described in the Guidelines document, focused on reliability. Reliability means that different people with different backgrounds that make an observation will see the same thing most of the time. To support the use of a clinical assessment, good-quality clinical studies must allow determination of the sensitivity, specificity, and the positive or negative predictive value of the test. For the purposes of the methods used in this document, the authors decided that the most important aspect of the clinical assessment test was its positive predictive value, or the number of patients who had the clinical sign or prognostic indicator and had a poor outcome. The authors arbitrarily decided that a recommendation for use of a clinical assessment test had to be supported by clinical studies that found a positive predictive value of 70% or greater.

These guidelines are divided into two sections: Assessment and Treatment and Hospital Transport Decisions. Conclusions regarding assessment tests, and

Table 3. Guidelines for Prehospital Management of Traumatic Brain Injury

a Assessment

	Diagnostic and prognostic value	Measurement
Oxygenation and blood pressure	Hypoxemia or hypotension are associated with poor outcome in the prehospital setting	*How to measure*: pulse oximeter for blood oxygenation; the most accurate method available for measurement of systolic and diastolic blood pressure *When to measure*: both should be measured as often as possible and monitored continuously if possible *Who should measure*: trained medical personnel
GCS score	The prehospital measurement of the GCS is a significant and reliable indicator of the severity of TBI, particularly in association with repeated scoring and improvement or deterioration of the score over time. A single field measurement of the GCS cannot predict outcome; however, a decrease of two points from a GCS of 9 or lower indicates serious injury. A score of 3–5 has at least a 70% positive predictive value for poor outcome	*How to measure*: the GCS must be obtained through interaction with the patient *When to measure*: after the initial assessment, a clear airway is established, and necessary ventilatory or circulatory resuscitation has been performed. It should be obtained prior to the administration of sedative or paralytic medications, or after these drugs have been metabolized *Who should measure*: trained emergency medical services personnel
Pupils	Insufficient data to support conclusions	*How to examine*: asymmetry is defined as a >1 mm difference in size; a fixed pupil is <1 mm response to bright light; evidence of orbital trauma should be noted; the presence and side of fixed and dilated pupils should be noted *When to examine*: after resuscitation and stabilization *Who should examine*: trained prehospital care providers

Table 3. (continued)

b Treatment, and Hospital Transport Decisions

	Standard	Guideline	Option
Airway, ventilation and oxygenation	None	Hypoxemia must be avoided, if possible, or corrected immediately. When equipment is available, oxygen saturation should be monitored for all patients as frequently as possible or continuously. Hypoxemia should be corrected by administering supplemental oxygen	The airway should be secured in patients who have a GCS <9, the inability to maintain an adequate airway, or hypoxemia not corrected by supplemental oxygen. Endotracheal intubation, if available, is the most effective procedure for this purpose. Routine prophylactic hyperventilation should be avoided. Hyperventilation in the field is indicated only when signs of cerebral herniation, such as extensor posturing or pupillary abnormalities, are present after correcting hypotension or hypoxemia. Normal ventilation is defined as approximately 10 breaths per minute for adults, 20 for children, and 30 for infants
Fluid resuscitation	None	Fluid resuscitation is essential to avoid hypotension and/or limit hypotension to the shortest duration possible. Hypotension is defined as a systolic blood pressure less than 65 mm Hg in infants, <75 for ages 2–5, <80 for ages 6–12, and <90 mm Hg for older children and adults	Isotonic saline is most commonly used for fluid resuscitation. Hypertonic saline may also be used, but no studies support the use of mannitol

Table 3. (continued)

b Treatment, and Hospital Transport Decisions

	Standard	Guideline	Option
Brain-targeted therapy	None	None	*Treatment of herniation*: hyperventilation is the first line of treatment. If effective in reversing the signs of herniation it should not be continued. Mannitol is not recommended *Treatment to optimize patient transport*: sedation, analgesia and neuromuscular blockade can be useful. The timing and choice of agents are best left to local EMS protocols *Treatment of other causes of altered mental status*: patients with altered mental status of undetermined etiology should have a rapid glucose determination, or be given glucose empirically
Hospital transport decisions	None	All regions should have an organized trauma care system that develops protocols to direct EMS personnel regarding transport of trauma victims. Recognizing at the scene or in the ambulance that a patient has a severe TBI guides hospital destination. Such patients should be transported directly to a facility that has immediately available CT, prompt neurosurgical care, and ability to monitor and treat ICP	All EMS systems should develop transport protocols to help make specific decisions regarding trauma center destinations for TBI patients. Patients with a GCS of 9–13 have the potential for intracranial injury and need for neurosurgical intervention, and should therefore be transported to a trauma center for evaluation

EMS = Emergency Medical Services.

recommendations regarding treatment or transport, are then provided for several specific topics considered most important in the prehospital setting. For the assessment guidelines, the diagnostic and prognostic value of assessment measures are provided as well as recommendations on how to measure it, when to measure it, and who should measure it. For the section on treatment and transport decisions, the 'standards, guidelines and options' format is utilized.

Guidelines for the Management of Penetrating Brain Injury

In 2001 guidelines entitled Management and Prognosis of Penetrating Brain Injury were published as a supplement to the *Journal of Trauma* [6] (table 4). The authors were Bizhan Aarabi, Tord D. Alden, Randall M. Chesnut, J. Hunter Downs 3rd, James M. Ecklund, Howard M. Eisenberg, Elana Farace, Robert E. Florin, John A. Jane, Jr., Mark D. Krieger, Andrew I.R. Maas, Raj K. Narayan, Alexander A. Potapov, Andres M. Salazar, Mark E. Shaffrey, and Beverly C. Walters. The format for development of these guidelines was similar to that used for the previous TBI guidelines documents. In addition to these treatment recommendations, the report also includes a section on prognostic indicators. The authors examined the relationship between Glasgow Coma Scale (GCS), pupil size and reactivity, age, hypotension and CT findings with outcome.

Pediatric Brain Injury

In 2003 the Guidelines for the Acute Management of Severe Traumatic Brain Injury in Infants, Children, and Adolescents were published as a supplement to *Pediatric Critical Care Medicine* [7] (table 5). Authors of this document were P. David Adelson, Susan L. Bratton, Nancy A. Carney, Randall M. Chesnut, Hugo E.M. du Coudray, Brahm Goldstein, Patrick M. Kochanek, Helen C. Miller, Michael D. Partington, Nathan R. Selden, Craig R. Warden, and David W. Wright. The methodology used for the development of these guidelines were the same as those used to develop the Guidelines for the Management of Severe Head Injury (Adults). Fifteen topics relevant to the acute care of children with severe TBI were addressed. These guidelines refer to children below the age of 18 years who have sustained a severe TBI and have a postresuscitation GCS of 3–8. They do not refer to victims of asphyxiation, drowning, or birth trauma. In the source document the authors also have included a comparison of their findings with those of the adult guidelines (Indications from Adult Guidelines) as a fourth entry in the Recommendations section. The document is otherwise written in a format very similar to the adult

Table 4. Guidelines for the Management of Penetrating Brain Injury [6]

	Standard	Guideline	Option
Neuroimaging	None	None	CT scanning of the head is strongly recommended. In addition to the standard axial views with bone and soft tissue windows, coronal sections may be helpful in patients with skull base or high convexity involvement. Plain radiographs of the head can be helpful in assessing bullet trajectory, the presence of large foreign bodies, and the presence of intracranial air. However, when CT scanning is available, plain radiographs are not essential and are not recommended as routine. Angiography is recommended when a vascular injury is suspected. Patients with an increased risk of vascular injury include cases in which the wound's trajectory passes through or near the Sylvian fissure, supraclinoid carotid, cavernous sinus, or a major venous sinus. The development of substantial and otherwise unexplained subarachnoid hemorrhage or delayed hematoma should also prompt consideration of a vascular injury and of angiography. Routine MRI is not generally recommended. MRI may have a role in evaluating injuries from penetrating wooden or other nonmagnetic objects. The utility of other imaging modalities such as intraoperative ultrasound, PET, SPECT, and image-guided stereotaxis has not yet been studied and recommendations cannot be made
ICP monitoring	None	None	Early ICP monitoring is recommended when the clinician is unable to assess the neurologic examination accurately, the need to evacuate a mass lesion is unclear, or imaging studies suggest elevated ICP. In the absence of studies specific to managing intracranial hypertension, we recommend that the clinician follow the recommendations of the Guidelines for the Management of Severe Traumatic Brain Injury
Surgical management	None	None	Treatment of small entrance bullet wounds to the head with local wound care and closure in patients whose scalp is not devitalized and have no 'significant' intracranial pathologic findings is recommended. (Note: The term 'significant' has

Table 4. (continued)

	Standard	Guideline	Option
			yet to be clearly defined. However, the volume and location of the brain injury, evidence of mass effect, e.g., displacement of the midline >5 mm or compression of basilar cisterns from edema or hematoma, and the patient's clinical condition, all pertain to significance.) Treatment of more extensive wounds associated with nonviable scalp, bone, or dura with more extensive debridement before primary closure or grafting to secure a watertight wound is recommended. In patients with significant fragmentation of the skull, debridement of the cranial wound with either craniectomy or craniotomy is recommended. In the presence of significant mass effect, debridement of necrotic brain tissue and safely accessible bone fragments is recommended. Evacuation of intracranial hematomas with significant mass effect is recommended. In the absence of significant mass effect, surgical debridement of the missile track in the brain is not recommended. Routine surgical removal of fragments lodged distant from the entry site and reoperation solely to remove retained bone or missile fragments are not recommended. Repair of an open-air sinus injury with a watertight dural closure is recommended. Clinical circumstances dictate the timing of the repair. Any repairs requiring duraplasty can be at the discretion of the surgeon as to material used for the closure
Vascular complications	None	None	CT angiography and/or conventional angiography should be considered to identify a traumatic intracranial aneurysm or arteriovenous fistula in patients with a penetrating brain injury involving an orbitofacial or pterional injury, particularly in patients harboring an intracerebral hematoma. When a traumatic intracranial aneurysm or arteriovenous fistula is identified, surgical or endovascular management is recommended
Cerebrospinal fluid leaks	None	None	Surgical correction is recommended for CSF leaks that do not close spontaneously, or are

Table 4. (continued)

	Standard	Guideline	Option
			refractory to temporary CSF diversion. During the primary surgery, every effort should be made to close the dura and prevent CSF leaks
Antibiotic prophylaxis	None	None	Use of prophylactic broad-spectrum antibiotics is recommended for patients with penetrating brain injuries
Antiseizure prophylaxis	None	None	Antiseizure medications in the first week after a penetrating brain injury are recommended to prevent early posttraumatic seizures. (e.g. phenytoin, carbamazepine, valproate, or phenobarbital). Prophylactic treatment beyond the first week has not been shown to prevent the development of new seizures, and is not recommended

Table 5. Guidelines for the Acute Management of Severe Traumatic Brain Injury in Infants, Children, and Adolescents [7]

	Standard	Guideline	Option
Trauma systems, pediatric trauma centers, and the neurosurgeon	None	In a metropolitan area, pediatric patients with severe TBI should be transported directly to a pediatric trauma center if available	Pediatric patients with severe TBI should be treated in a pediatric trauma center or in an adult trauma center with added qualifications to treat children in preference to a level I or II adult trauma center without added qualifications for pediatric treatment
Prehospital airway management	None	Hypoxia must be avoided if possible and attempts made to correct it immediately. Supplemental oxygen should be administered. There is no evidence to support an advantage of endotracheal intubation over bag-valve-mask ventilation	If prehospital endotracheal intubation is instituted for pediatric TBI patients, then specialized training and use of end-tidal CO_2 detectors is necessary

Table 5. (continued)

	Standard	Guideline	Option
Resuscitation of blood pressure and oxygenation and prehospital brain-specific therapies	None	Hypotension should be identified and corrected as rapidly as possible with fluid resuscitation. In children, hypotension is defined as a systolic blood pressure below the fifth percentile for age or by clinical signs of shock. Tables depicting normal values for pediatric blood pressure by age are available. Evaluation for associated extracranial injuries is indicated in the setting of hypotension	Airway control should be obtained in children with a GCS <9 to avoid hypoxemia, hypercarbia, and aspiration. Initial therapy with 100% O_2 is appropriate in the resuscitation phase of care. Oxygenation and ventilation should be assessed continuously by pulse oxymetry and end-tidal CO_2 monitoring, respectively, or by serial blood gas measurements. Hypoxia should be identified and corrected rapidly. Blood pressure should be monitored frequently and accurately. Fluids should be administered to maintain the blood pressure in the normal range. Sedation, analgesia, and neuromuscular blockade can be useful to optimize transport of the patient. The prophylactic administration of mannitol is not recommended. Mild prophylactic hyperventilation is not recommended
Indications for ICP monitoring	None	None	ICP monitoring is appropriate in infants and children with severe TBI. The presence of open fontanels and/or sutures in an infant with severe TBI does not preclude the development of ICH or negate the utility of ICP monitoring. ICP monitoring is not routinely indicated in infants and children with mild or moderate head injury
Threshold for treatment of ICP	None	None	Treatment for ICH should begin at an ICP >20 mm Hg. Interpretation and treatment of ICH based on any ICP threshold should be corroborated by frequent clinical examination, monitoring of physiologic variables, and cranial imaging
ICP monitoring technology	None	None	A ventricular catheter or an external strain gauge transducer or catheter tip pressure

Table 5. (continued)

	Standard	Guideline	Option
			transducer device is an accurate and reliable method of monitoring ICP. A ventriculostomy catheter device also enables therapeutic CSF drainage
Cerebral perfusion pressure	None	A CPP >40 mm Hg should be maintained	A CPP between 40 and 65 mm Hg probably represents an age-related continuum for the optimal treatment threshold. There may be exceptions to this range in some infants and neonates. Advanced cerebral physiologic monitoring may be useful to define the optimal CPP in individual instances. Hypotension should be avoided
Sedation and neuromuscular blockade	None	None	The choice and dosing of sedatives, analgesics, and neuromuscular blocking agents should be left to the treating physician. However, the effect of individual sedatives and analgesics on ICP can be variable and unpredictable
Role of CSF drainage	None	None	CSF drainage can be considered as an option in the management of elevated ICP. Drainage can be accomplished via a ventriculostomy catheter alone or in combination with a lumbar drain. The addition of lumbar drainage should be considered as an option only in the case of refractory ICH with a functioning ventriculostomy, open basal cisterns, and no evidence of a major mass lesion of shift on imaging studies
Hyperosmolar therapy	None	None	Hypertonic saline and mannitol are effective for control of ICH. Euvolemia should be maintained by fluid replacement. A Foley catheter is recommended. Serum osmolarity should be maintained below 320 mosm/l with mannitol use, whereas a level of 360 mosm/l appears to be tolerated with hypertonic saline. The choice of mannitol or hypertonic saline as a first-line hyperosmolar agent should be left to the treating physician

Table 5. (continued)

	Standard	Guideline	Option
Hyperventilation	None	None	Mild or prophylactic hyperventilation ($PaCO_2$ <35 mm Hg) should be avoided. Mild hyperventilation may be considered for longer periods for ICH refractory to sedation and analgesia, neuromuscular blockade, CSF drainage, and hyperosmolar therapy. Aggressive hyperventilation ($PaCO_2$ <30 mm Hg) may be considered as a second tier option in the setting of refractory ICH. CBF, jugular venous O_2 saturation, or brain tissue O_2 monitoring is suggested to help identify cerebral ischemia in this setting. Aggressive hyperventilation therapy titrated to clinical effect may be necessary for brief periods in cases of cerebral herniation or acute neurologic deterioration
Barbiturates	None	None	High-dose barbiturate therapy may be considered in hemodynamically stable patients with salvageable severe TBI and refractory ICH. If used, appropriate hemodynamic monitoring and cardiovascular support are essential
Temperature control	None	None	Extrapolated from adult data, hyperthermia should be avoided. Despite the lack of clinical data in children, hypothermia may be considered in the setting of refractory ICH
Surgical treatment	None	None	Decompressive craniectomy should be considered when there is diffuse cerebral swelling and ICH refractory to intensive medical management, particularly in those children with abusive head trauma if they are considered to have a potentially recoverable brain injury
Corticosteroids	None	None	Steroids are not recommended for improving outcome or reducing ICP

CBF = Cerebral blood flow; CPP = cerebral perfusion pressure; ICH = intracranial hypertension.

guidelines, and includes overview, process, scientific foundation, summary, and key issues for future investigation sections. For each topic the search strategies are clearly described, and evidentiary tables are included.

Guidelines for the Surgical Management of Severe Traumatic Brain Injury

This document has been submitted for publication. The authors are Ross M. Bullock, Randall Chesnut, Jamshid Ghajar, David Gordon, Roger Hartl, David W. Newell, Franco Servadei, Beverly C. Walters, and Jack Wilberger, and production of the document was supported by the Brain Trauma Foundation (table 6). For these guidelines the authors focused on three issues that were considered most relevant for deciding whether or not to operate: indications for surgery, timing, and the type of operation (method).

Why Are There So Few Standards?

Four of the Guidelines documents summarized above contain recommendations for specific treatments classified as standards, guidelines, or options, based on the strength of the evidence supporting the recommendation. The four documents list a total of 38 treatment recommendations, but in only 3 of those recommendations was there evidence sufficient to support recommending the treatment as a standard. All three of the standards are in the Guidelines for the Management of Severe Traumatic Brain Injury, and recommend against the use of treatments: prophylactic hyperventilation, steroids, and anticonvulsants. No treatment standards could be recommended for any of the pediatric, prehospital, or penetrating TBI guidelines. And evidence sufficient to support recommendations at the level of a guideline was available for only 16 of the 38 topics.

In defining which treatments for severe TBI were supported by class I evidence, (standards) and which were not, a goal of the original Guidelines workgroup was to determine which treatments needed to be tested in prospective randomized clinical trials. In this and the subsequent Guidelines documents, a section entitled 'Key Issues for Future Investigation' was included at the end of each chapter to provide details for what the authors thought was needed to establish a standard for a particular diagnostic test or therapy. It was hoped that such explicit direction would lead to numerous clinical trials that would provide the class I evidence needed to elevate guidelines or options to standards. But such research has not been forthcoming.

Table 6. Surgical Management of Traumatic Brain Injury

	Indications for surgery	Timing	Methods
Acute epidural hematomas	An epidural hematoma >30 ml should be surgically evacuated regardless of the patient's GCS. An epidural hematoma <30 ml and with <15 mm thickness and with <5 mm midline shift in patients with a GCS >8 without focal deficit can be managed nonoperatively with serial CT scanning and close neurologic observation in a neurosurgical center	It is strongly recommended that patients with an acute epidural hematoma in coma with anisocoria undergo surgical evacuation as soon as possible	There are insufficient data to support one surgical treatment method. However, craniotomy provides a more complete evacuation of the hematoma
Acute subdural hematomas	An acute subdural hematoma with a thickness >10 mm or midline shift >5 mm on CT should be surgically evacuated, regardless of the patient's GCS. All patients with an acute subdural hematoma in coma should undergo ICP monitoring. A comatose patient with a subdural hematoma <10 mm thickness and midline shift <5 mm should undergo surgical evacuation of the lesion if the GCS decreases between the time of injury and hospital admission by 2 or more points and/or the patient presents with asymmetric or fixed and dilated pupils and/or the ICP exceeds 20 mm Hg	In patients with acute subdural hematoma and indications for surgery, surgical evacuation should be done as soon as possible	If surgical evacuation of an acute SDH in a comatose patient is indicated, it should be done using a craniotomy with or without bone flap removal and duraplasty
Traumatic parenchymal lesions	Patients with parenchymal mass lesions and signs of progressive neurologic deterioration referable to the lesion, medically refractory intracranial hypertension, or signs of mass effect on CT scan should be treated operatively. Patients with GCS of 6–8 with frontal or temporal contusions greater than 20 ml in volume with midline shift >4 mm and/or cisternal compression on CT scan, and patients with any lesion greater than 50 ml in volume, should be treated operatively. Patients with parenchymal mass lesions who do not show evidence for	Bifrontal decompressive craniectomy within 48 h of injury is a treatment option for patients with diffuse, medically refractory posttraumatic cerebral edema and resultant intracranial hypertension	Craniotomy with evacuation of mass lesion is recommended for those patients with focal lesions and the surgical indications listed above. Decompressive procedures, including subtemporal decompression, temporal lobectomy and hemispheric decompressive craniectomy, are

Table 6. (continued)

	Indications for surgery	Timing	Methods
	neurologic compromise have controlled ICP, and no significant signs of mass effect on CT scan may be managed nonoperatively with intensive monitoring and serial imaging		treatment options for patients with refractory intracranial hypertension and diffuse parenchymal injury with clinical and radiographic evidence for impending transtentorial herniation
Posterior fossa mass lesions	Patients with mass effect on CT scan or with neurologic dysfunction or deterioration referable to the lesion should undergo operative intervention. Mass effect on CT scan is defined as distortion, dislocation, or obliteration of the fourth ventricle, compression or loss of visualization of the basal cisterns, or the presence of obstructive hydrocephalus. Patients with lesions and no significant mass effect on CT scan who have no signs of neurologic dysfunction may be managed by close observation and serial imaging	In patients with indications for surgical intervention, evacuation should be performed as soon as possible since these patients can deteriorate rapidly, thus worsening their prognosis	Suboccipital craniectomy is the predominant method reported for evacuation of posterior fossa mass lesions, and is therefore recommended
Depressed skull fractures	Patients with open (compound) skull fractures depressed greater than the thickness of the skull should undergo operative intervention to prevent infection. Such patients may be treated nonoperatively if there is no clinical or radiographic evidence of dural penetration, significant intracranial hematoma, depression >1 cm, frontal sinus involvement, gross cosmetic deformity, wound infection, pneumocephalus, or gross wound contamination. Nonoperative management of closed (simple) depressed skull fractures is a treatment option	Early operation is recommended to reduce the incidence of infection	Elevation and debridement are recommended as the surgical method of choice. Primary bone fragment replacement is a surgical option in the absence of wound infection at the time of surgery. All management strategies for open depressed fractures should include antibiotics

There are several reasons why investigators have been reluctant to conduct the research prescribed in the Guidelines documents. The most common is a strong clinical bias: clinical experience and/or a preponderance of basic science evidence supports the use of a particular treatment or diagnostic test. As a result, many clinicians consider unethical a randomized clinical trial in which half the patients would not receive the treatment or diagnostic test. The following fall into this category:

- Blood pressure resuscitation (measurement of the effect of hypotension)
- ICP (measurement of the effect of intracranial hypertension)
- Mannitol
- Nutrition (measurement of the effect of withholding nutritional supplementation)
- Physiologic monitoring such as blood pressure, ICP (measure the effect of treatment without monitoring)

A second problem is the cost of doing clinical trials for TBI. Most trauma centers admit less than 40 patients with severe TBI/year. Clinical TBI trials with adequate power usually require 400 or more subjects, so either a large number of contributing centers must be included, or the trial must extend for a prohibitive period of time. The most commonly accepted outcome measure is the Glasgow Outcome Scale score obtained at 6 months after injury. However, the accurate, timely, and independent measurement of 6-month outcomes is very expensive. Unless money is available for tracking study subjects and traveling when necessary to test them, unacceptably high attrition rates undermine the conclusions of the study. These and other issues have led many to believe that the clinical trials needed to elevate options and guidelines to standards are unlikely to be done.

Evidence that Guidelines for the Management of Severe Traumatic Brain Injury Have Influenced Outcomes

Since publication of the original Guidelines document several studies have examined changes in practice as a result of the Guidelines, and the impact of the Guidelines on outcomes following severe TBI. A survey of North American neurosurgeons published in 2000 queried these individuals about their use of specific treatments that were discussed in the Guidelines document [8]. Compared to a survey published in 1995 [1], the responding neurosurgeons indicated that there was a 55% increase in the use of ICP monitoring, a 47% decrease in the use of prophylactic hyperventilation therapy, and a 45% decrease in the use of steroids.

Recent studies also suggest that the Guidelines have led to improved outcomes [9–13]. The most important of these studies was published by Fakhry et al. [9] in the March 2004 issue of the *Journal of Trauma*. It describes the outcomes for 830 patients with severe TBI who were cared for either before, during, or after institution of evidence-based guidelines at the Inova Fairfax Hospital in Falls Church, Va., USA. During 1991–1994 (before guidelines) 219 patients with severe TBI were admitted. Guidelines were introduced in 1995–1996 but there was poor compliance, and during that time 188 patients with severe TBI were admitted. From 1997 to 2000 compliance with the guidelines was high, and during that time 423 patients with severe TBI were admitted. The admission GCS score for the 'before guidelines group' was slightly higher than for the other two groups, but in every other way the three groups were similar. Compared to the before guidelines group, the 'after guidelines group' had a shorter ICU stay by 1.8 days, and shorter length of stay in the acute care hospital by 5.4 days, in both cases statistically significant differences. The mortality rate for the after guidelines group was 4% lower that for the before guidelines group. The good recovery rate (mild, moderate or no disability at discharge) for the after guidelines group was 61.5% compared to 43.3% for the before guidelines group, also a statistically significant difference. To control for general improvements in critical care over this 10-year span, the authors studied similar outcomes in a group of 1,060 trauma patients that did not have TBI who were treated at their hospital from 1991 to 2000. Demographics and injury severity scores were similar except for the absence of TBI. During this period of time the ICU length of stay actually increased by 3.5 days, and the length of acute care hospitalization and mortality rates remained the same for the trauma patients without head injuries. The authors therefore concluded that improved outcomes for patients with severe TBI most likely were the result of the implementation and use of evidence-based guidelines. Similar conclusions were derived from a study of 93 TBI patients published by Palmer et al. [10]. They compared outcomes for 37 patients treated before implementation of the Guidelines with the outcomes for 56 patients treated after they began using the Guidelines. They found that implementation of the Guidelines led to a 9.13 times higher odds ratio of a good outcome.

It might be expected that the impact of a particular set of guidelines on practice would be diminished in inverse proportion to the weight of evidence supporting the recommendations. However, it appears that the documents have provided a basis on which to develop consistent treatment protocols at individual hospitals [14–16]. This trend alone has been an important step forward and helps to improve the care provided to TBI patients.

References

1 Ghajar J, Hariri RJ, Narayan RK, et al: Survey of critical care management of comatose, head-injured patients in the United States. Crit Care Med 1995;23:560–567.

2 US Department of Health and Human Services. Interagency Head Injury Task Force Report. Washington, US Department of Health and Human Services, 1989.
3 Bullock R, Chesnut RM, Clifton G, Ghajar J, Marion DW, Narayan RK, Newell DW, Pitts LH, Rosner MJ, Walters BC, Wilberger JE: Guidelines for the management of severe head injury. J Neurotrauma 1996;13:638–817.
4 Brain Trauma Foundation: American Association of Neurological Surgeons and Joint Section on Neurotrauma and Critical Care: Guidelines for the management of severe traumatic brain injury, and early prognostic indicators of prognosis in severe traumatic brain injury. J Neurotrauma 2000;17:451–627.
5 Gabriel EJ, Ghajar J, Jagoda A, Pons PT, Scalea T, Walters BC; Brain Trauma Foundation: Guidelines for prehospital management of traumatic brain injury. J Neurotrauma 2002;19:111–174.
6 Pruitt BA Jr: Management and prognosis of penetrating brain injury. J Trauma 2001;51(suppl 2): S1–S86.
7 Adelson PD, Bratton SL, Carney NA, Chesnut RM, du Coudray HE, Goldstein B, Kochanek PM, Miller HC, Partington MP, Selden NR, Warden CR, Wright DW; American Association for Surgery of Trauma; Child Neurology Society; International Society for Pediatric Neurosurgery; International Trauma Anesthesia and Critical Care Society; Society of Critical Care Medicine; World Federation of Pediatric Intensive and Critical Care Societies: Guidelines for the acute medical management of severe traumatic brain injury in infants, children, and adolescents. Pediatr Crit Care Med 2003;4(3 suppl):S1–S71.
8 Marion DW, Spiegel TP: Changes in the management of severe traumatic brain injury: 1991–1997. Crit Care Med 2000;28:16–18.
9 Fakhry SM, Trask AL, Waller MA, Watts DD; IRTC Neurotrauma Task Force: Management of brain-injured patients by an evidence-based medicine protocol improves outcomes and decreases hospital charges. J Trauma 2004;56:492–499.
10 Palmer S, Bader MK, Qureshi A, Palmer J, Shaver T, Borzatta M, Stalcup C: The impact on outcomes in a community hospital setting of using the AANS traumatic brain injury guidelines. Americans Associations for Neurologic Surgeons. J Trauma 2001;50:657–664
11 Naredi S, Koskinen LO, Grande PO, Nordstrom CH, Nellgard B, Rydenhag B, Vegfors M: Treatment of traumatic head injury – U.S./European guidelines or the Lund concept. Crit Care Med 2003;31:2713–2714.
12 Citerio G, Stocchetti N, Cormio M, Beretta L, Galli D, Pesenti A: Application of guidelines for severe head trauma: data from an Italian database. Eur J Emerg Med 2003;10:68–72.
13 Bulger EM, Nathens AB, Rivara FP, Moore M, MacKenzie EJ, Jurkovich GJ; Brain Trauma Foundation: Management of severe head injury: institutional variations in care and effect on outcome. Crit Care Med 2002;30:1870–1876.
14 Mcilvoy L, Spain DA, Raque G, Vitaz T, Boaz P, Meyer K: Successful incorporation of the Severe Head Injury Guidelines into a phased-outcome clinical pathway. J Neurosci Nurs 2001;33:72–78, 82.
15 Sesperez J, Wilson S, Jalaludin B, Seger M, Sugrue M: Trauma case management and clinical pathways: prospective evaluation of their effect on selected patient outcomes in five key trauma conditions. J Trauma 2001;50:643–649.
16 Littlejohns LR, Bader MK: Guidelines for the management of severe head injury: clinical application and changes in practice. Crit Care Nurse 2001;21:48–65.

Donald W. Marion, MD
35 High Rock Road
Wayland, MA 01778 (USA)
Tel. +1 508 358 4551, Fax +1 508 358 5510, E-Mail donmarion1@yahoo.com

Pollock BE (ed): Guiding Neurosurgery by Evidence.
Prog Neurol Surg. Basel, Karger, 2006, vol 19, pp 197–207

Treatment of Chronic Pain with Neurostimulation

John K. Birknes, Ashwini Sharan, Ali R. Rezai

Departments of Neurosurgery and Neurology, Thomas Jefferson University, Philadelphia, Pa., USA

Abstract

Chronic pain conditions are a complex and multifactorial problem generally requiring a multidisciplinary-type approach. The central nervous system at some point clearly becomes involved in the processing of these painful conditions with an integration of complex changes in neurophysiology and behavior. Many ablative techniques have been employed in the past to interrupt these signals. However, the results were often temporary and symptoms tended to recur. The more modern approach has suggested that modulation of the nervous elements may be a more resilient approach for treating such chronic pain disorders. We are realizing that many of these pain conditions are also dynamic and evolving, and as such need a similar treatment modality. Neurostimulation, thus, provides the ability of therapeutically dosing electrical current in a variety of pulse forms, amplitudes, pulse widths, and frequencies, to affect that system. Furthermore, it is not destructive, it is reversible, and it can be remotely adjusted and programmed over time; clear advantages to previous surgical therapies. This chapter reports on the current evidence for the use of neurostimulation (i.e. spinal cord stimulation, motor cortex stimulation and deep brain stimulation) in the treatment of chronic pain conditions.

The therapeutic use of electrical stimulation for pain relief is an ancient art. The Egyptians and the Greeks used electric eels to apply shock therapy and the Romans applied the torpedo fish to treat maladies such as cephalgia and arthralgia [1–3].

Subsequently, the modern learning elucidated the anatomy of the pain tracts and it became evident that electrical stimulation of the nervous system could be predictably used for therapeutic benefits. In the mid 1900s, neurosurgeons were routinely applying electrical stimulation to the brain to treat and to study movement, psychiatric and pain disorders. In fact in 1954, Heath [4] and Pool [5] both reported on implantation of temporary electrodes in the septum pellucidum to treat patients with schizophrenia and pain from metastatic carcinoma. Many other targets have since been enthusiastically explored for the treatment of patients with chronic pain including the thalamus, caudate, cingulate, or periaqueductal grey. With the renewed interest in chronic deep brain stimulation (DBS), it is hopeful that physicians may again study and offer patients an opportunity to interrupt the pain circuits in the deep cerebral targets.

The further use of central nervous system stimulation developed with the introduction of the gate theory for pain control by Melzack and Wall [6]. They noted that stimulation of large myelinated fibers of peripheral nerves resulting in paresthesias blocked the activity in small nociceptive projections. Shealy [7] and Shealy and Cady [8] applied this knowledge in 1967 by inserting the first dorsal column stimulator in a human suffering from terminal metastatic cancer. The therapeutic use of electrical stimulation developed further when Shealy, in collaboration with Long, prompted Hagfers and Maurer to independently produce the first two solid state transcutaneous electrical nerve stimulators [7, 8]. (Actually, transcutaneous electrical nerve stimulators were originally developed as a screening tool for spinal cord stimulators.) Subsequently, electrodes have been implanted via a laminectomy in the subarachnoid space, between the two layers of the dura or in the epidural space, both dorsal or ventral to the spinal cord and later the percutaneous technique was introduced [9–14]. More recently motor cortex stimulation (MCS) as well as DBS have been used in the treatment of various pain conditions.

Chronic pain conditions are becoming an increasing problem with growing costs generally requiring a multidisciplinary-type approach. The central nervous system at some point clearly becomes involved in the processing of these painful conditions with an integration of complex changes in neurophysiology and behavior. Many ablative techniques have been employed in the past to interrupt these signals. However, the results were often temporary and they tended to recur.

The more modern approach has suggested that modulation of the nervous elements may be a more resilient approach for treating such chronic pain disorders. We are realizing that many of these pain conditions are also dynamic and evolving, and as such need a similar treatment modality. Neurostimulation, thus, provides the ability of therapeutically dosing electrical current in a variety of pulse forms, amplitudes, pulse widths, and frequencies, to affect that system. Furthermore, it is not destructive, it is reversible, and it can be remotely adjusted and programmed over time. These are clear advantages to previous surgical therapies.

Spinal Cord Stimulation

Spinal cord stimulation (SCS) has been utilized for a variety of pain conditions. The most common indications include failed back surgery syndrome (FBSS), complex regional pain syndrome (CRPS), ischemic limb pain, and angina. SCS is particularly indicated with any type of 'neuropathic' pain. Indications have been extended to cover the treatment of intractable pain due to other causes including cervical neuritis pain, spinal cord injury pain, postherpetic neuralgia, neurogenic thoracic outlet syndrome, and temporomandibular joint syndrome refractory to multiple surgical interventions.

Although a large body of work has been published, the exact mechanisms of action of SCS remain unclear. The computer modeling work of Coburn and colleagues [15–17] and, more recently, of Holsheimer and colleagues [18–20] has shed some light, at least theoretically, on the distribution of the electrical fields within the spinal structures. It is clear that stimulation on the dorsal aspect of the epidural space creates complex electrical fields which affect a large number of structures. We do not know whether activating afferents within the peripheral nerve, dorsal columns, or supralemniscal pathways share equivalent mechanisms of action. Additionally, there may be antidromic action potentials passing caudally in the dorsal columns to activate spinal segmental mechanisms in the dorsal horns as well as action potentials ascending in the dorsal columns activating cells in the brainstem, which in turn might activate descending inhibition. At the chemical level, animal studies suggest that the SCS triggers the release of serotonin, substance P, and GABA within the dorsal horn [21–23].

Failed Back Surgery Syndrome

Two prospective controlled studies were found. Marchand et al. [24] examined patients who had undergone at least one prior surgery for chronic back pain secondary to trauma. Each of these patients was currently using an SCS and they acted as their own controls. Eight patients participated in 4 testing sessions each (2 sets of 2). In the first set of 2 sessions noxious stimulation and analgesia were tested; during one session the stimulator was on the patient's normal settings while during the other session it was nonfunctional. The second set of two sessions evaluated discrimination of visual and noxious heat stimuli with the stimulator on for one session and off for the other. Pain scores were significantly reduced with SCS compared to placebo stimulation.

North et al. [25] conducted a prospective study randomizing patients with FBSS. One group underwent repeat back surgery while the other underwent SCS surgery. All patients presented with standard clinical and radiographic criteria for surgical intervention. After 6 months, patients were permitted to cross over to the alternative therapy if they were dissatisfied with their results. Ten of 15 patients crossed over from back surgery to SCS (67%), while only 2 of 12 patients crossed over from SCS to back surgery (17%; $p = 0.018$).

Eight other prospective studies reporting on over 300 patients exist on SCS for back and leg pain [26–33]. When including all studies (retrospective, prospective with and without controls) successful treatment of FBSS with SCS was observed in 62% of patients ($n = 747$). Successful treatment was defined as greater than 50% reduction in pain or significant reduction in visual analogue scale (VAS) score [34].

CRPS I and II

CRPS I is also known as reflex sympathetic dystrophy. One prospective controlled study and three prospective studies without matched controls were found in the literature. Kemler et al. [35] examined 54 patients with CRPS I (reflex sympathetic dystrophy) and randomized them, using a 2:1 ratio, to receive either SCS with physical therapy (PT; $n = 36$) or PT alone ($n = 18$). Twenty-four of the 36 (67%) patients in the SCS group experienced significant relief with percutaneous stimulation and thus received a permanent implant. The remaining 12 patients did not undergo surgery but their data was included in the SCS group in the final analysis.

Pain and quality of life measurements were obtained at 1, 3 and 6 months. At 6 months a significant improvement was demonstrated in the SCS group with the VAS reduced by 2.4 cm compared with a 0.2-cm increase in the PT group ($p < 0.0001$). No functional improvement was observed in either group. With long-term follow-up at 2 years, this significance was unchanged with a VAS reduction in SCS group of 2.1 cm and a 0-cm change in the PT group.

Three prospective studies without matched controls were discovered (total of 50 subjects) [36–38]. Two of the studies reported success rates with an 84% overall success rate. The third study by Calvillo et al. [38] reported a significant improvement in pain scores (VAS) and a >50% reduction in narcotic use by 44% of subjects. In eight retrospective studies the overall success rate was 84% (192 patients) [34].

Ischemic Limb Pain

Two controlled prospective randomized studies exist. Klomp et al. [39] randomized 120 patients, with critical painful limb ischemia, to receive either best medical therapy alone or SCS in conjunction with best medical therapy. At a mean follow-up of 19 months, there was no significant difference in pain score improvement between the two groups. The SCS group did, however, report a significant reduction in pain medication in the short term. Jivegard et al. [40] authored a similar study where 51 patients were randomized to receive either oral medication alone or SCS with oral medication. Conversely, they reported a significant improvement in pain scores of the SCS-treated group over the non-SCS group ($p < 0.01$).

Four prospective studies without matched controls [41–44] in the literature reveal an overall success rate of 78% ($n = 271$). Analysis of seven retrospective studies found an overall success rate of 76% ($n = 308$) [34].

Angina Pain

Three prospective controlled studies in the literature address SCS for angina. Hautvast et al. [45] implanted an SCS in patients with stable angina pectoris and randomized them. One group's SCS was inactivated while the other group was instructed to use the stimulator 3 times per day for 1 h and with any angina attack. At 6 weeks, a significant reduction in both the number of angina attacks and nitrate consumption was observed in the functioning SCS group. Additionally these patients exhibited an increased exercise duration.

Mannheimer et al. [46] randomized 104 patients accepted for coronary artery bypass graft (CABG) to receive either CABG ($n = 51$) or SCS ($n = 53$). Both groups experienced a significant reduction in both the number of angina attacks and the consumption of nitrates. There was no significant intergroup difference regarding these parameters. Interestingly the CABG group was found to have a significantly higher mortality rate.

De Jongste et al. [47] randomized 17 patients with angina to an active treatment group (i.e. SCS implantation) and a control group. The control group was followed for 2 months, at the end of which period, they too received SCS implantation. Both groups were followed for a total of 12 months. This study also revealed a significant reduction in the incidence of angina attacks and in the consumption of nitrates ($p < 0.05$).

Five additional studies are reported to be prospective but without matched controls [48–52]. Each of these revealed significant benefit from spinal cord stimulation. The benefit indices ranged from reduction in angina attacks, decrease nitrate consumption, decrease in NYHA grade and improvement in NHP grade.

MCS/Precentral Stimulation

In 1991, Tsubokawa et al. [53] first reported on their experience using epidural MCS to treat 12 patients with deafferentation pain. A chronic stimulating electrode was placed epidurally such that stimulation of the underlying cortex produced motor contractions in the painful region. Experimental work by Tsubokawa et al. [54–56] demonstrated that thalamic hyperactivity could be reduced by chronic sensorimotor cortex stimulation and this established the foundation for the clinical treatment. Since then, many other groups have independently reported on the treatment of chronic pain conditions via cortical targets [57–71].

The central idea underlying the therapeutic effect of MCS is activation of nonnociceptive sensory neurons which are believed to exert an inhibitory effect on their nociceptive counterparts. This type of interaction may be present at multiple levels of the somatosensory pathway along the peripheral and central nervous systems. Further, induction of motor contractions in the area of the pain often may result in pain relief.

As is true with most therapies available for these different chronic pain conditions, the results vary tremendously and depend largely on the differing definitions of success. MCS has been most consistently used for trigeminal neuropathic pain and poststroke or central pain. Nguyen et al. [72–74] reported on 22 patients with trigeminal pain where 13 obtained marked improvement and 5 obtained satisfactory improvement. Only 4 were not improved. Ebel et al. [75] reported sustained good to excellent relief in 3 of 7 patients over time with trigeminal pain. Meyerson et al. [64] have reported between 60 and 90% pain relief on 5 patients with trigeminal neuropathic pain. Tsubokawa et al. [53] initially reported on the treatment of central pain with MCS with 8 of 12 patients having continued effect after 1 year of therapy. Many others have reported on their experience with similar patients. Katayama et al. [63] noted satisfactory results in 2 of 3 patients with brainstem infarcts. Mertens et al. [76] also noted 60% excellent or good relief in poststroke pain. An analysis of the literature by Nguyen et al. [72] has revealed 52% success (82 of 159 patients) for central pain. Expert opinion suggests a role of MCS for neuropathic trigeminal pain and poststroke pain [77].

Presently, there are no prospective trials using MCS and there are only 23 major cases series reported in the literature [77]. The largest case series included 32 patients and the majority of reports include less than 10 subjects. In general, the body of literature regarding this technique is plagued by a lack of controlled and blinded studies, a lack of uniformly classified diseases, and reporting on a small series of patients. However, the world experience with this therapy still remains young but standardization of the technique will likely bear out its merits in time.

Deep Brain Stimulation

As previously mentioned, Heath [4] and Pool [5] in 1954 both reported on the implantation of temporary electrodes in the septum pellucidum to treat patients with schizophrenia and pain from metastatic carcinoma. The technique of DBS was then described in the ventroposterolateral thalamic nucleus by

Mazars et al. [78] in 1960. Other targets were subsequently explored. Periaqueductal gray and periventricular gray matter (PAG/PVG) stimulation was described by multiple groups [79–81].

The exact mechanism of pain modulation by DBS is unknown. PAG/PVG stimulation is, however, felt to result in stimulation of an opioid-dependent pathway. Thalamic stimulation may modulate the abnormal firing patterns in the thalamic neurons secondary to deafferentation.

Currently, the two most common targets for DBS for pain include the periventricular grey matter or the ventrocaudalis thalamus. As a generalization, patients with neuropathic pain should undergo paresthesia-producing stimulation with implantation in ventrocaudal (Vc) thalamus while those patients with nociceptive pain should undergo PAG/PVG stimulation. Many patients will inevitably have mixed components of nociceptive and neuropathic pain and thus both Vc and PAG/PVG stimulation trials may be indicated. The internal capsule and medial lemniscus have also been successfully used.

Since the therapy of DBS for pain has been practiced for decades, many case series have been published [81–89]. It seems that patients with nociceptive pain as in cancer pain and FBSS respond best to DBS. Published series of PAG/PVG stimulation have reported treatment of cancer pain and FBSS with success rates ranging from 25 to 100% and 30 to 80%, respectively. Additionally, brachial plexus injuries, peripheral neuropathies, and phantom limb pain appear to respond to Vc DBS. Although the use of DBS for chronic pain precedes SCS and MCS, no prospective study has evaluated its use.

Conclusion

The treatment of chronic pain remains difficult. Neurostimulation for chronic pain is definitely a treatment option. There is currently insufficient class 1 evidence available to assess the full benefits of SCS, MCS, and DBS. All three therapies have reported around 50% relief of pain. Future studies will have to be designed with randomization of patients, placebo or sham stimulation, and uniformity in terms of classification of pain types before full understanding and defining of the benefits of each modality.

References

1 Stillings D: A survey of the history of electrical stimulation for pain to 1900. Med Instrum 1975;9:255–259.

2 Kellaway P: The part played by electric fish in the early history of bioelectricity and electrotherapy. Bull Hist Med 1946;20:112–137.

3 Schiller F: The history of algology, algotherapy, and the role of inhibition. Hist Philos Life Sci 1990;12:27–50.

4 Heath R: Studies in Schizophrenia: a Multidisciplinary Approach to Mind-Brain Relationships. Cambridge, Harvard University Press, 1954.

5 Pool J: Psychosurgery in older people. J Am Geriatr Soc 1954;2:456–465.

6 Melzack R, Wall P: Pain mechanisms: a new theory. Science 1965;150:971–979.

7 Shealy CN: Dorsal column stimulation: optimization of application. Surg Neurol 1975;4:142–145.

8 Shealy C, Cady R: Historical perspective of pain management; in Weiner RS (ed): Pain Management: a Practical Guide for Clinicians. Boca Raton, St Lucie Press, 1998, pp 7–15.

9 Hoppenstein R: Electrical stimulation of the ventral and dorsal columns of the spinal cord for relief of chronic intractable pain. Surg Neurol 1975;4:187–194.

10 Larson S, Sances A, Cusick J, Meyer G, Swiontek T: A comparison between anterior and posterior implant systems. Surg Neurol 1975;4:180–186.

11 Larson SJ, Sances A Jr, Riegel DH, Meyer GA, Dallmann DE, Swiontek T: Neurophysiological effects of dorsal column stimulation in man and monkey. J Neurosurg 1974;41:217–223.

12 Lazorthes Y, Verdie J, Arbus L: Stimulation analgésique médullaire antérieure et postérieure par technique d'implantation percutanée. Acta Neurochir 1978;40:253–276.

13 Dooley DM: Spinal cord stimulation. AORN J 1976;23:1209–1212.

14 Dooley D: Percutaneous electrical stimulation of the spinal cord. Assoc Neurol Surg, Bal Harbour, 1975.

15 Coburn B: Electrical stimulation of the spinal cord: two-dimensional finite element analysis with particular reference to epidural electrodes. Med Biol Eng Comput 1980;18:573–584.

16 Coburn B: A theoretical study of epidural electrical stimulation of the spinal cord. II. Effects on long myelinated fibers. IEEE Trans Biomed Eng 1985;32:978–986.

17 Coburn B, Sin WK: A theoretical study of epidural electrical stimulation of the spinal cord. I. Finite element analysis of stimulus fields. IEEE Trans Biomed Eng 1985;32:971–977.

18 Holsheimer J, Struijk JJ: How do geometric factors influence epidural spinal cord stimulation? A quantitative analysis by computer modeling. Stereotact Funct Neurosurg 1991;56:234–249.

19 Holsheimer J, Barolat G, Struijk JJ, He J: Significance of the spinal cord position in spinal cord stimulation. Acta Neurochir Suppl 1995;64:119–124.

20 Holsheimer J, Wesselink WA: Effect of anode-cathode configuration on paresthesia coverage in spinal cord stimulation. Neurosurgery 1997;41:654–660.

21 Linderoth B, Stiller CO, Gunasekera L, O'Connor WT, Ungerstedt U, Brodin E: Gamma-aminobutyric acid is released in the dorsal horn by electrical spinal cord stimulation: an in vivo microdialysis study in the rat. Neurosurgery 1994;34:484–489.

22 Linderoth B: Dorsal column stimulation and pain: experimental studies of putative neurochemical and neurophysiological mechanisms. Stockholm, Kongl Carolinska Medico Chirurgiska Institutet, 1992.

23 Foreman RD, Beall JE, Coulter JD, Willis WD: Effects of dorsal column stimulation on primate spinothalamic tract neurons. J Neurophysiol 1976;39:534–546.

24 Marchand S, Bushnell MC, Molina-Negro P: The effects of dorsal column stimulation on measures of clinical and experimental pain in man. Pain 1991;45:249–257.

25 North RB, Kidd D, Piantadosi S: Spinal cord stimulation versus reoperation for failed back surgery syndrome: a prospective, randomized study design. Acta Neurochir Suppl (Wien) 1995;64: 106–108.

26 Leibrock LG, Meilman P, Cuka D, et al: Spinal cord stimulation in the treatment of chronic back and lower extremity pain syndromes. Nebr Med J 1984;69:180–183.

27 LeDoux MS, Langford KH: Spinal cord stimulation for the failed back syndrome. Spine 1993;18:191–194.

28 Burchiel KJ, Anderson VC, Brown FD, et al: Prospective, multicenter study of spinal cord stimulation for relief of chronic back and extremity pain. Spine 1996;21:2786–2793.

29 Barolat G, Oakley JC, Law JD, et al: Epidural spinal cord stimulation with a multiple electrode paddle lead is effective in treating intractable low back pain. Neuromodulation 2001;4:59–66.

30 Kavar B, Rosenfeld JV, Hutchinson A: The efficacy of spinal cord stimulation for chronic pain. J Clin Neurosci 2000;7:409–413.

31 Ohnmeiss DD, Rashbaum RF, Bogdanffy GM: Prospective outcome evaluation of spinal cord stimulation in patients with intractable leg pain. Spine 1996;21:1344–1351.
32 Shatin D, Mullett K, Hults G: Totally implantable spinal cord stimulation for chronic pain: design and efficacy. Pacing Clin Electrophysiol 1986;9:577–583.
33 Rainov NG, Heidecke V, Burkert W: Short test-period spinal cord stimulation for failed back surgery syndrome. Minim Invasive Neurosurg 1996;39:41–44.
34 Cameron T: Safety and efficacy of spinal cord stimulation for the treatment of chronic pain: a 20-year literature review. J Neurosurg Spine 2004;100:254–267.
35 Kemler MA, Barendse GA, Van Kleef M: Spinal cord stimulation in patients with chronic reflex sympathetic dystrophy. N Engl J Med 2000;343:618–624.
36 Ebel H, Balogh A, Volz M: Augmentative treatment of chronic deafferentation pain syndromes after peripheral nerve lesions. Minim Invasive Neurosurg 2000;43:44–50.
37 Oakley J, Weiner RL: Spinal cord stimulation for complex regional pain syndrome: a prospective study of 19 patients at 2 centers. Neuromodulation 1999;2:47–50.
38 Calvillo O, Racz G, Didie J, et al: Neuroaugmentation in the treatment of complex regional pain syndrome of the upper extremity. Acta Orthop Belg 1998;64:57–63.
39 Klomp HM, Spincemaille GH, Steyerberg EW: Spinal-cord stimulation in critical limb ischaemia: a randomised trial. ESES Study Group. Lancet 1999;353:1040–1044.
40 Jivegard LEH, Augustinsson LE, Holm J: Effects of spinal cord stimulation (SCS) in patients with inoperable severe lower limb ischaemia: a prospective randomised controlled study. J Vasc Endovasc Surg 1995;9:421–425.
41 Graber JN, Lifson A: The use of spinal cord stimulation for severe limb-threatening ischemia: a preliminary report. Ann Vasc Surg 1987;1:578–582.
42 Horsch S, Claeys L: Epidural spinal cord stimulation in the treatment of severe peripheral arterial occlusive disease. Ann Vasc Surg 1994;8:468–474.
43 Rickman S, Wuebbels BH, Holloway GA Jr: Spinal cord stimulation for relief of ischemic pain in end-stage arterial occlusive disease. J Vasc Nurs 1994;12:14–20.
44 Petrakis E, Sciacca V: Spinal cord stimulation in critical limb ischemia of the lower extremities: our experience. J Neurosurg Sci 1999;43:285–293.
45 Hautvast RW, DeJongste MJ, Staal MJ: Spinal cord stimulation in chronic intractable angina pectoris: a randomized, controlled efficacy study. Am Heart J 1998;136:1114–1120.
46 Mannheimer C, Eliasson T, Augustinsson L: Electrical stimulation versus coronary artery bypass surgery in severe angina pectoris: the ESBY study. Circulation 1998;97:1157–1163.
47 de Jongste MJL, Hautvast RWM, Hillege HL: Efficacy of spinal cord stimulation as adjuvant therapy for intractable angina pectoris: a prospective, randomized clinical study. Working Group on Neuroradiology. J Am Coll Cardiol 1994;23:1592–1597.
48 Eliasson T, Jern S, Augustinsson L, et al: Safety aspects of spinal cord stimulation in severe angina pectoris. Coron Artery Dis 1994;5:845–850.
49 Sanderson JE, Ibrahim B, Waterhouse D, et al: Spinal electrical stimulation for intractable angina – long-term clinical outcome and safety. Eur Heart J 1994;15:810–814.
50 Andersen C: Complications in spinal cord stimulation for treatment of angina pectoris. Differences in unipolar and multipolar percutaneous inserted electrodes. Acta Cardiol 1997;52:325–333.
51 Bagger JP, Jensen BS, Johannsen G: Long-term outcome of spinal cord electrical stimulation in patients with refractory chest pain. Clin Cardiol 1998;21:286–288.
52 Vulink NCC, Overgaauw DM, Jessurun GAJ, et al: The effects of spinal cord stimulation on quality of life in patients with therapeutically chronic refractory angina pectoris. Neuromodulation 1999;2:33–40.
53 Tsubokawa T, Katayama Y, Yamamoto T, Hirayama T, Koyama S: Chronic motor cortex stimulation for the treatment of central pain. Acta Neurochir Suppl (Wien) 1991;52:137–139.
54 Tsubokawa T, Katayama Y, Yamamoto T, Hirayama T, Koyama S: Chronic motor cortex stimulation in patients with thalamic pain. J Neurosurg 1993;78:393–401.
55 Tsubokawa T, Katayama Y, Yamamoto T, Hirayama T, Koyama S: Treatment of thalamic pain by chronic motor cortex stimulation. Pacing Clin Electrophysiol 1991;14:131–134.
56 Tsubokawa T, Katayama Y: Motor cortex stimulation in persistent pain management; in Gildenberg PL, Tasker RR (eds): Textbook of Stereotactic and Functional Neurosurgery. New York, McGraw Hill, 1998, pp 1547–1556.

57 Canavero S, Bonicalzi V, Castellano G, Perozzo P, Massa-Micon B: Painful supernumerary phantom arm following motor cortex stimulation for central poststroke pain. Case report. J Neurosurg 1999;91:121–123.
58 Canavero S, Bonicalzi V: Cortical stimulation for central pain. J Neurosurg 1995;83:1117.
59 Ebel H, Rust D, Tronnier V, Boker D, Kunze S: Chronic precentral stimulation in trigeminal neuropathic pain. Acta Neurochir Suppl (Wien) 1996;138:1300–1306.
60 Franzini A, Ferroli P, Servello D, Broggi G: Reversal of thalamic hand syndrome by long-term motor cortex stimulation. J Neurosurg 2000;93:873–875.
61 Fujii M, Ohmoto Y, Kitahara T, Sugiyama S, Uesugi S, Yamashita T, Shiroyama Y, Ito H: Motor cortex stimulation therapy in patients with thalamic pain (in Japanese). No Shinkei Geka 1997;25: 315–319.
62 Hosobuchi Y: Motor cortical stimulation for control of central deafferentation pain. Adv Neurol 1993;63:215–217.
63 Katayama Y, Tsubokawa T, Yamamoto T: Chronic motor cortex stimulation for central deafferentation pain: experience with bulbar pain secondary to Wallenberg syndrome. Stereotact Funct Neurosurg 1994;62:295–299.
64 Meyerson BA, Lindblom U, Linderoth B, Lind G, Herregodts P: Motor cortex stimulation as treatment of trigeminal neuropathic pain. Acta Neurochir Suppl (Wien) 1993;58:150–153.
65 Nguyen JP, Keravel Y, Feve A, Uchiyama T, Cesaro P, Le Guerinel C, Pollin B: Treatment of deafferentation pain by chronic stimulation of the motor cortex: report of a series of 20 cases. Acta Neurochir Suppl 1997;68:54–60.
66 Nguyen JP, Lefaucher JP, Le Guerinel C, Eizenbaum JF, Nakano N, Carpentier A, Brugieres P, Pollin B, Rostaing S, Keravel Y: Motor cortex stimulation in the treatment of central and neuropathic pain. Arch Med Res 2000;31:263–265.
67 Rainov NG, Fels C, Heidecke V, Burkert W: Epidural electrical stimulation of the motor cortex in patients with facial neuralgia. Clin Neurol Neurosurg 1997;99:205–209.
68 Roux FE, Ibarrola D, Lazorthes Y, Berry I: Chronic motor cortex stimulation for phantom limb pain: a functional magnetic resonance imaging study: technical case report. Neurosurgery 2001;48:681–688.
69 Saitoh Y, Shibata M, Hirano S, Hirata M, Mashimo T, Yoshimine T: Motor cortex stimulation for central and peripheral deafferentation pain. Report of eight cases. J Neurosurg 2000;92:150–155.
70 Nandi D, Smith H, Owen S, Joint C, Stein J, Aziz T: Peri-ventricular grey stimulation versus motor cortex stimulation for post stroke neuropathic pain. J Clin Neurosci 2002;9:557–561.
71 Yamamoto T, Katayama Y, Hirayama T, Tsubokawa T: Pharmacological classification of central post-stroke pain: comparison with the results of chronic motor cortex stimulation therapy. Pain 1997;72:5–12.
72 Nguyen J, Lefaucheur J, Keravel Y: Motor cortex stimulation; in Burchiel K (ed): Electrical Stimulation and the Relief of Pain. Amsterdam, Elsevier Science, 2003, pp 197–209.
73 Nguyen J, Keravel Y, Feve A, et al: Treatment of deafferentation pain by chronic stimulation of the motor cortex: report of a series of 20 cases. Acta Neurochir Suppl 1997;68:54–60.
74 Nguyen JP: Motor cortex stimulation. 10th World Congress on Pain, San Diego, 2002.
75 Ebel H, Rust D, Tronnier V, et al: Chronic precentral stimulation in trigeminal neuropathic pain. Acta Neurochir Suppl (Wien) 1996;138:1300–1306.
76 Mertens P, Nuti C, Sindou M, et al: Precentral cortex stimulation for the treatment of central neuropathic pain. Stereotact Funct Neurosurg 1999;73:122–125.
77 Sharan AD, Rosenow JM, Turbay M, Testerman R, Rezai AR: Precentral stimulation for chronic pain. Neurosurg Clin N Am 2003;14:1–7.
78 Mazars G, Roge R, Mazars Y: Stimulation of the spinothalamic fasciculus and their bearing on the pathophysiology of pain. Rev Neurol 1960;103:136–138.
79 Richardson D, Akil H: Pain reduction by electrical brain stimulation in man. 1. Acute administration in periaqueductal and periventricular sites. J Neurosurg 1977;47:178–183.
80 Richardson D, Akil H: Pain reduction by electrical brain stimulation in man. 2. Chronic self-administration in the periventricular gray matter. J Neurosurg 1977;47:184–194.
81 Hosobuchi Y, Adams J, Linchitz R: Pain relief by electrical stimulation of the central gray matter in humans and its reversal by naloxone. Science 1977;197:183–186.

82 Richardson D, Akil H: Long term results of periventricular gray self-stimulation. Neurosurgery 1977;1:199–202.
83 Young R, Kroening R, Fulton W, et al: Electrical stimulation of the brain in treatment of chronic pain. J Neurosurg 1985;62:389–396.
84 Turnball I, Shulman R, Woodhusst W: Thalamic stimulation for neuropathic pain. J Neurosurg 1980;52:486–493.
85 Meyerson B, Boethius J, Carlsson A: Alleviation of malignant pain by electrical stimulation in the periventricular region: pain relief as related to stimulation sites. Adv Pain Res Ther 1979;3: 525–533.
86 Levy R, Lamb S, Adams J: Treatment of chronic pain by deep brain stimulation: long term follow-up and review of the literature. Neurosurgery 1987;21:885–893.
87 Kumar K, Toth C, Nath R: Deep brain stimulation for intractable pain: a 15-year experience. Neurosurgery 1997;40:736–746.
88 Tasker R, Vilela Filho O: Deep brain stimulation for neuropathic pain. Stereotact Funct Neurosurg 1995;65:122–124.
89 Dieckmann G, Witzmann A: Initial and long-term results of deep brain stimulation for chronic intractable pain. Appl Neurophys 1982;45:167–172.

Ashwini D. Sharan, MD
Assistant Professor of Neurosurgery and Neurology
Thomas Jefferson University
909 Walnut Street, 3rd Floor
Philadelphia, PA 19107 (USA)
Tel. +1 215 955 7000, Fax +1 215 503 7007

Author Index

Subject Index